More My ᴍᴏʟᴀʀ Pregnancy

Personal Stories From Diagnosis Through Recovery

Edited by

Jennifer Wood Gilbreath

All of the medical information in this book is given either as a general overview or as individual descriptions of personal experiences. It should not be used for diagnostic or treatment purposes. For all medical concerns and questions, please contact your physician. I am not responsible for problems arising from the misuse of this material.

The stories in this second volume were collected in late 2012 and early 2013, although when the authors' original experiences occurred varies widely. Requests for submissions were placed on several Facebook Groups, including the two MyMolarPregnancy support groups, and the related Facebook page. All of the authors have granted permission for the use of their stories in this collection, with the understanding that they retain the right to share their stories elsewhere. I only retain copyright of the printed versions as they appear in this publication.

Anyone wishing to reprint this text in part or whole in any format should contact me by e-mail at mymolarpregnancy@gmail.com.

For additional stories, information, links, and support for molar pregnancy, visit http://www.mymolarpregnancy.com.

From my darkness came my Sunshine.
Without the shadows,
I would never have had the light.

Contents

Foreword

Gestational trophoblastic disease (called GTD) is a rare group of interrelated tumors that develop following conception that is caused by abnormal development of the placenta. More than eighty percent of GTD cases are molar pregnancies, a form of miscarriage that is non-cancerous. The malignant forms of GTD called invasive mole and choriocarcinoma can be treated, and in the great majority of cases the treatment results in a cure.

Most women who have had a single incidence of GTD can go on to have normal pregnancies. This was not the case before 1956 when a group of investigators at the National Cancer Institute first used methotrexate to treat a woman with malignant GTD that had spread throughout her body. Prior to that time, women who developed GTD which was still localized to the uterus (called non-metastatic) could be cured with hysterectomy, with loss of reproductive function. Once the disease traveled from the uterus to other organs (called metastatic), however, it was usually fatal.

The idea to use methotrexate to treat this disease was inspired by the observation of an obscure clinician, MC Li, at Memorial Sloan-Kettering Institute in New York City who observed that a positive pregnancy test turned negative after a female patient with liver cancer received methotrexate, one of the few chemotherapy agents available at that time. Methotrexate had been used successfully before in treating acute childhood leukemia at Boston's Children's Hospital by Dr. Sidney Farber. But this is the first time it showed that it could be used in the treatment of patients with solid tumors. MC Li brought this observation with him when he joined Dr. Roy Hertz and the team at the National Cancer Institute. Dr. Hertz, a distinguished endocrinologist, for many years had been working on the interaction of folic acid and cell growth. They reasoned that if methotrexate which blocked the production of folic acid, could kill the cells in the liver cancer that were making the pregnancy hormone, human chorionic gonadotropin (also called hCG), that it might also be used to kill choriocarcinoma and other forms of gestational trophoblastic disease that also produce high levels of hCG.

Through trial and error the dosage to be used and the frequency of administration were painstakingly developed so that by 1963 the group at the National Cancer Institute was able to report that nearly half of the first sixty-three cases treated were cured. This report galvanized the oncology community and encouraged Congress to provide support for the development of the field of medical oncology. Part of this support was directed to establish treatment centers for GTD at Harvard, Duke and Northwestern where it was demonstrated that patients treated at Trophoblastic Disease Centers had improved survival.

Over the past sixty years enormous progress has been made in our understanding of the incidence and causes of this condition and in its management. In the United States there are approximately sixty-five hundred cases annually of benign GTD (molar pregnancy) of which approximately twenty percent develop malignancy and require treatment. Worldwide it is estimated that there are two hundred thousand cases of molar pregnancy annually. GTD also rarely develops following normal childbirth and miscarriage. Treatment centers have now been established in many developed and developing nations. Other drugs have been introduced to treat patients that do not respond to methotrexate. The roles of other treatment modalities, such as surgery and radiation, have also been defined. In contrast to the pre-chemotherapy era, all patients whose disease is localized to the uterus and most patients with metastatic disease can now be cured with PRESERVATION OF REPRODUCTIVE FUNCTION.

Jennifer Wood's monograph *My Molar Pregnancy* is a collection of personal stories from patients who were diagnosed and treated for gestational trophoblastic disease. It vividly portrays the other aspect of this disease, its emotional impact on the patient, her spouse, her family, and her friends. As physicians we tend to be focused on the mechanics of treating the disease, making sure we're using the right drugs, doses, time intervals and watching for serious side effects. What we don't see is how this disease and its treatment impacts on the patient after she leaves our office. *My Molar Pregnancy* helps women confront and deal with the fears, concerns, and questions that this diagnosis raises and makes us realize how important it is to understand the personal as well as the medical issues. What comes through loud and clear, in addition to the trials and tribulations of treatment, is the deep sadness and disappointment associated with loss of the pregnancy that leads to the disease.

I strongly recommend this book to all women with GTD because it will help them and their families understand both its emotional and medical aspects.

Donald Peter Goldstein, M.D.
New England Trophoblastic Disease Center
Division of Gynecologic Oncology
Dana Farber/Brigham and Women's Cancer Center
Harvard Medical School
Boston, Massachusetts

Preface

In 2013 I was in an accident and sustained a brain injury that required a great deal of recovery time. My son, Xander, lives with his father since our divorce; Xander is autistic, and his father, Jason, is a special education teacher, so we had decided it was the best situation for him. Because of my injury and inability to handle Xander on my own, I saw him infrequently in the first few months of my recovery. After several months, however, I was finally able to begin driving, working from home, and could at last see my son without assistance. I still wasn't able to return to a regular job and work schedule, so I even got to see Xander more than I had before the accident, because I was no longer fettered by the busy work schedule I'd had since the divorce. I finally had time to be "Mommy" again, something I had missed terribly.

My time was short lived, however. In January 2014, Jason told me that circumstances with his family and his wife's family up north were making it necessary for them to move back there to be closer to them. Unable to support Xander or handle his autism myself, and knowing he would be better off with more family and the better school and community supports up there than in Florida, I reluctantly agreed to let him go with them. When they moved in June, six months later, I kept Xander with me and my husband Bill for a week before we took him to his new home. I knew it was the right decision, and that he would have more support, more family, and more educational opportunities there—all the things a mother wants for her child. Nonetheless, driving my son one thousand miles north and leaving him behind ripped my heart out just as painfully as that day in April 2001 when the doctor told me there was no baby inside me. My dream—of what was to be, of how life was going to be, of what was to come, of what was *supposed* to happen—had been ruined. Without Bill to support me, I don't know how I would have gotten through what I felt as another loss. Yes, I was able to see Xander six months later at Christmas, but those six months, counting out the months and weeks and days, were like the year of waiting after my molar diagnosis: time passing while your life is in limbo. For me, once again, my Xander—my rainbow baby—was waiting for me at the end of it. I had come full circle.

Why am I telling you all this? What I'm trying to say is, life is a roller coaster that twists and turns and lifts and drops and never seems to end, always sending you in unexpected directions. As you ride, you see glimpses of the tracks you have already ridden, the good and the bad, as they flash past you, and you are reminded of the feelings, the cheering highs or the stomach-sinking lows, that those moments held for you. If you've recently been diagnosed with a molar pregnancy, then right now you are quite possibly sinking into one of those lows, dropping fast and feeling as though you will never come back up. Molar pregnancy is nearly impossible to comprehend. Hearing that diagnosis for the first time and the explanation of what is happening to you is like having the ultimate experience of vertigo. The ceiling spins, your brain reels, and your stomach lurches like a sudden short lift and drop in the coaster.

No one should be alone on a ride like that, and I hope that each and every person reading this book has someone, a partner, a family member, a friend—someone with whom they can talk about their feelings, share their experience and grief, explore their questions, and look forward to their future. This book, the book that came before it, my website, and the support groups that I operate are all here for you in addition to your someone—or even if no one else is there for you. Often others won't understand what you are going through, and that is not their fault; they simply can't relate. There are people out there who can. Find them. The Internet has made the world a much smaller place, and you can find what you need if you take the time to look. You are reading this book, so you have taken a huge step already; if you go online and join our support groups you may just meet some of these amazing ladies "in person" online or others like them who have been where you are.

The "Introduction" that follows is very similar to the one from the previous collection, with only a few updates and changes, because all of the basics—my background, the history of the website, information about molar pregnancy, and so on—were covered there already. That does not mean you shouldn't take a look at the first book if you haven't already; there are at least thirty more stories there, including my own in full detail, which I have not included here. I had hoped to have this book out much earlier than this; my 2013 accident took me out of the loop for a while, so I thank all of the contributors for their patience.

To all of you reading this book, I hope you find what you are looking for, whether it is peace and understanding for yourself, a better understanding of molar pregnancy for a loved one, or just a casual interest in this little known condition. I am sorry for your loss, and I wish you health and happiness in the future.

Acknowledgements

I have to thank all of the women who have passed through my support groups over these past fourteen(!) years for all of the work they have done supporting each other. You come in hurt and grieving and afraid, and then you stay and learn and support the next group. That is what makes it work.

My heartfelt thanks to Drs. Goldstein and Berkowitz of the New England Trophoblastic Disease Center at Dana Farber/ Brigham and Women's Cancer Center in Boston, Massachusetts.

The work you and your team do helps so many, and your incredible kindness to patients, both those under your direct care and those who contact you from the outside in search of help and answers, is felt deeply by all of us. I am also incredibly grateful to Stacey Katz Friedlander, who has tirelessly worked to raise awareness and funds for both Brigham and Women's Cancer Center and MyMolarPregnancy.com by organizing an annual National Gestational Trophoblastic Disease Awareness Day Walk/Run/Ride and other events. Your efforts are admirable and appreciated.

Dad and Momma: I love you, and I have never doubted that you love me, no matter what else. Thank you for that.

Bill, you pull me out of my box and make me try, do, taste, and experience new things that I never would have done without your encouragement. Thank you for making me—I mean, giving me the opportunity to—photograph alligators from an inflatable kayak ten feet away and swim springs and climb waterfalls and mountains. I love you.

Xander, you are my everything. There is nothing on this Earth that I would not do for you. I do not know how much you will ever understand all of this, but I want you to know that as sad as I was to lose that first baby, I know that it's because I was meant to be *your* mommy. I love you bigger than the sky. You make me proud every single day, my beautiful boy.

Jason and Carolyn: I trust you with my most precious gem in the universe. Thank you for guarding him with such care and love.

Introduction

I founded MyMolarPregnancy in June 2001, just six weeks after my own diagnosis. Confused and grieving, I had searched the Internet for information about the condition and what it meant for me in both the near and distant future. I was angry, and hurting, and jealous of all the other pregnant women around me. I needed to find someone who could understand what I was feeling and offer comfort and support. No one in my family or among my friends had ever heard of a molar pregnancy, and they could not comprehend the fear I was feeling in addition to the grief of losing a baby. After a while, many of them thought I should be "getting over it" and moving on, but I was trapped in a year-long limbo of waiting and wondering. Would this be the month my levels go up? Would I ever get pregnant again? Was I capable of having a normal pregnancy? What was my risk of cancer, or of having another mole? At the doctor's office, the nurses who saw the elevated hCG levels in my chart assumed I was pregnant and coming in for a prenatal checkup. Time and again I had to tell them I wasn't pregnant anymore. Then I usually had to explain the entire mess all over again to convince them. My husband was supportive, but he was grieving and scared as well. He didn't want to talk about it. I felt so alone and needed so badly to share those feelings.

The first incarnation of the MyMolarPregnancy site went live on June 14, 2001. It consisted of a page or two with my story, some links and information, a guestbook, and an online support group. Within a few weeks I had nearly twenty members in the group. I soon made friends with several women in varying stages of the process. We shared our fears and grief as well as our frustration with our doctors. We learned that treatment approaches varied considerably from coast to coast and around the globe. Members began doing their own Internet research and coming to the group with new articles or information they'd found. It was the beginning of the healing process for me. I was sharing my pain with people who understood, and at the same time I was taking this horrible experience and turning it something useful that could help others. In February 2002 I purchased the MyMolarPregnancy.com domain name, and my little page became a full-fledged website. I began adding personal stories submitted by other women as well, because although we share a common diagnosis and a common loss, each of us has had different experiences. Some have had chemotherapy; some have gone on to successful pregnancies. Some had their molar pregnancies long ago, some are still having their blood tests monthly, and some are just receiving their diagnoses.

I have heard so many stories, some inspiring and others devastating, but all of them familiar. This book and the one that came before it are my way of reaching out beyond the Internet to reach the women who—for whatever reason—are unable or unwilling to share their grief online but who still need the kind of support that can be found only by connecting with others who share the same experiences. Here you will find complete stories from nearly two dozen women who have been through the entire molar pregnancy experience, from diagnosis to treatment, through chemotherapy, and onward. Some, like me, have gone on to have happy, healthy pregnancies. Others have not. I won't promise you that every story has a happy ending. I can't say for certain what your future holds. But I believe that most women facing a molar pregnancy diagnosis will find a story in this book that they can relate to, and knowing you are not alone is the first step toward healing.

This book is about the subjective, personal, intimate experience of molar pregnancy. My knowledge of molar pregnancies comes mainly from my own experiences, those of the women I have met online in the past fourteen years, and the research I have found online. However, it is my hope that this book will be of use not only to women with molar pregnancies but also to their doctors, their friends, and their family members. To that end, I offer the following brief description of molar pregnancies and their treatment as well as suggestions for how friends, family members, doctors, and medical personnel can best approach and support a patient with molar pregnancy to ensure the best possible outcome. I am not a physician or scientist. The information that follows is intended to give you a general idea of what a molar pregnancy is, how it is treated, and what to expect from this diagnosis.

Gestational Trophoblastic Disease

Gestational trophoblastic disease, or GTD, also known as *gestational trophoblastic neoplasia,* is an umbrella term for molar pregnancy and its related forms, including complete, partial, invasive, and persistent mole; choriocarcinoma; and placental site trophoblastic tumor.

Complete Molar Pregnancy

There are two kinds of molar pregnancy. In a *complete molar pregnancy,* there is no genetic information in the fertilized egg, so the body has only the sperm's genes from which to develop a fetus. Essentially, the sperm fertilizes an "empty egg." Nonetheless, tissue begins to grow, usually appearing on ultrasound images as black circles often described as a "cluster of grapes." I saw this "cluster" on my own ultrasound. Left untreated, the tissue will continue to grow rapidly. It triggers the pregnancy hormone, known as *human chorionic gonadotropin,* or *hCG,* and seems to feed off it, increasing hCG levels exponentially. It is not uncommon for women who are only a few weeks along with a molar pregnancy to have hCG levels in the hundred-thousands, far beyond the levels expected in a normal pregnancy. This tissue grows and grows and can, in rare cases, develop into a cancerous malignancy known as *choriocarcinoma*. Upon diagnosis, molar tissue is generally removed immediately by *dilation and curettage (D&C)* to reduce or eliminate the risk of cancer. In the case of a complete mole, there has been no actual fetus, so removal is generally done right away with little consideration.

Partial Molar Pregnancy

The second kind of molar pregnancy is a *partial molar pregnancy*. In a partial mole, two sperm fertilize the same egg. Under normal circumstances this could lead to twins, and indeed many cases of partial molar pregnancy involve twin fetuses. However, in the case of a partial mole, the fetus(es) usually has too many chromosomes and eventually dies. It's not clear why this happens. Partial molar pregnancies are especially difficult because in many cases the mother has had at least one successful ultrasound and seen evidence of a heartbeat or other fetal development. I have even heard stories from women pregnant with twins for whom one twin has been viable and the other molar, leaving these mothers with the horrible choice of whether to terminate the pregnancy or risk cancer for the sake of the viable twin. Eventually, in most cases, the partial mole is removed by D&C, although some physicians have given patients the option to wait for a natural miscarriage. In other cases, such as those involving a viable twin, a wait-and-see approach is sometimes taken, depending on the risk to the mother.

Removal and Treatment

The standard procedure to remove molar tissue is a D&C, although as I mentioned there are some cases in which a woman is given the option to wait for natural miscarriage. In other cases women miscarry naturally without knowing they have had a molar pregnancy and are diagnosed much later and only after having reproductive problems that require an ultrasound or other testing. I won't go into specifics of the D&C procedure here. However, after the procedure, which is most often done on an outpatient basis, the woman usually is permitted to go home and recuperate. Over the next few days she must have blood drawn repeatedly, and a test known as a *beta quant* will be run on the samples to measure the level of hCG in her blood. It is important that the levels decline rapidly and continue to do so until returning to normal, nonpregnant levels, generally considered to be a level less than 5 (in some areas a level less than 2 is required). This may take several weeks, but the initial daily bloodwork will be cut back to weekly draws during that time as long as the hCG levels are declining. The woman's menstrual cycle may return during this time as well; my periods resumed eight weeks to the day after my D&C, but other women have had their periods return sooner and others much later. The first few periods may also be unusual—heavier than usual, off schedule, more or less crampy than usual, and so on—as the woman's body recovers.

If all goes well, the woman's hCG level should decline rapidly at first, then slower as she approaches a normal level, finally reaching normal several weeks after the D&C or miscarriage. Once a woman's hCG level reaches normal levels, the treatment approaches vary from doctor to doctor, region to region, and around the world. In the United States, for example, hCG is almost always measured in blood samples. However, in the United Kingdom and other parts of the world, urine samples are used. It is generally recommended that the woman be monitored for a period of time after the diagnosis to ensure that the hCG levels do not rise again. An increase in hCG would indicate that the molar tissue either has regrown or was not completely removed with the first procedure. Thus it is essential to monitor these levels for signs of regrowth. Because hCG is the "pregnancy hormone"—the hormone used to detect a pregnancy—the woman is instructed not to get pregnant during the monitoring period. This is for her safety, but it is often the source of much grief, anger, and frustration for the woman and her partner, especially if the woman's age or other medical conditions may affect her ability to get pregnant at a later time.

The standard monitoring period in the United States until recently has been twelve months for a woman with a complete molar pregnancy and six months for a woman with a partial mole. However, this varies considerably, and research over the past decade has caused some change in regular practice recommendations. I believe the current standard is three months' wait once hCG levels have returned to normal for a partial molar pregnancy; possibly longer for a complete molar or if any other issues or conditions arise. Remember, I'm not a doctor, so please don't take this as the rule, just what I see most often among women in my support groups these days. A great deal of research is available online, much of it dealing with the appropriate periods of monitoring. However, the ultimate decision should be left up to the woman and her doctor. Individual women's cases may have particular conditions that require longer-than-usual waiting times. I do not recommend women cut short their waiting period without at least discussing it with their physicians.

In addition to blood testing, women may also be referred for a chest X-ray at the time of their diagnosis. This is not a standard procedure, but it is often done to provide a baseline image, or starting image, in the event that the molar tissue becomes cancerous and metastasizes to the lungs.

Persistent and Invasive Moles

When moles regrow after the D&C, they are considered *persistent*. Often a second and even a third D&C may be done to try to remove the tissue, and this may be successful. However, in many cases the tissue continues to grow. If the mole grows into or beyond the uterus, or *metastasizes*, it is then classified as an *invasive mole*. Persistent and invasive moles must be chemically removed with chemotherapy. Please note that being treated with chemotherapy does not necessarily mean you have cancer. Chemotherapy is designed to kill targeted tissue, and that is what is needed in this situation. Methotrexate is the most frequently used chemotherapy drug for molar tissue, but there are others as well. The chemotherapy will be administered and then the woman's hCG levels will be monitored to see if they decrease. If they do not decline, more rounds of chemotherapy with the same or another drug may be necessary. The survival rate for women with moles that regrow within the uterus is 100 percent, and the survival rate for those whose moles metastasize to other body parts is 97 percent to 100 percent (Johnson and Schwartz 2007).

Choriocarcinoma

Choriocarcinoma is a malignant, cancerous form of GTD. It is an aggressive cancer that can rapidly spread to other parts of the body. However, it responds well to chemotherapy and has a survival rate of 75 percent to 100 percent depending on the situation (Johnson and Schwartz 2007).

Placental Site Trophoblastic Tumor

Placental site trophoblastic tumor is also a cancerous form of GTD. These tumors grow inside the uterus and do not involve hCG, therefore they are detected through visual imaging procedures such as magnetic resonance imaging (MRI) or ultrasound rather than through bloodwork and hCG measurements. The tumors generally do not spread beyond the uterus, but they are not responsive to chemotherapy, thus a hysterectomy is usually performed to remove them. The survival rate varies from 20 percent to 100 percent depending on when the tumor is first diagnosed (Johnson and Schwartz 2007).

The Experience of Being Diagnosed

One of biggest complaints I have heard from women with molar pregnancies relates to their treatment by the doctors, nurses, and ultrasound and laboratory technicians involved in making the initial diagnosis and overseeing the monitoring period. In my own experience I was evaluated by a nurse practitioner who, on seeing the molar cells on my ultrasound, blurted out, "20 percent of all pregnancies end in miscarriage!" and then bolted from the room, leaving my husband and me in shock. She offered no words of comfort or even to prepare us for the devastating news. The ultrasound technician who did my second ultrasound was not permitted to tell us anything of what she saw, but her face was grim, and her deep, painful movements with the ultrasound wand drove the bad news home nonetheless.

Lost in a sea of confusion and misinformation, I spent three days alternating between hopeful optimism and crushing despair. No one even told me about the chance of developing cancer from this condition; I found that out on the Internet! As I was wheeled out of surgery after my D&C, sobbing hysterically, one nurse admonished me for my tears and told me I was young, I'd have another baby soon; in fact, I was just a baby myself (I was twenty-six). Going back to my doctor's office for checkups in the weeks that followed, I often had to explain my condition to nurses who assumed I was there for a prenatal checkup because my bloodwork showed elevated levels of hCG. None of people charged with my care seemed to comprehend the vast range of feelings I was experiencing. I had lost a baby, yes, and they had seen other patients with miscarriages before, but they looked at me as though I was being overly dramatic when I explained there was more to it, that I was facing a chance of developing cancer, and that I did not appreciate being treated like a happy pregnant woman when I was grieving and afraid!

A woman who miscarries a pregnancy feels a devastating loss. She is left with questions and doubts: Why did it happen? Did I do something wrong? Will I be able to conceive again? Will I ever carry a baby to term? Family and friends flock around her and her partner offering sympathy and support as they grieve and begin the healing process. In most instances, the woman is told she can try again in three months or even sooner. Her time of waiting and healing is painful and difficult to be sure, but it passes, and the friends and family who saw her through it are still there to encourage her as she and her partner try again. It is generally expected (however unrealistically) that the partners will soon accept their loss and move onward with their lives.

For the woman who has lost a pregnancy to a mole, however, the loss of the baby is compounded by the risk of molar regrowth, the chance of developing cancer, and the requirement that the woman not get pregnant again for months, even as long as a year. The woman in her late childbearing years who receives this diagnosis is faced with the possibility of never having children. The same may be said for women who have had multiple "natural" miscarriages and have undergone expensive fertility treatments or for those who have developed additional reproductive complications, such as endometriosis or polycystic ovary syndrome. Even for the young and otherwise healthy woman who has plenty of childbearing years ahead, the diagnosis and the required monitoring time represent a period of limbo during which she must put all of her life plans on hold while waiting to see what will happen next. For all of these women the fear of regrowth and the risk of cancer weigh heavily on their hearts and minds. Days and weeks and months of blood tests leave them feeling like pin cushions and laboratory rats. While dealing with their own fear and grief, they often also must deal with doctors who have rarely or never treated a patient with molar pregnancy, medical staff who misread their charts, and family and friends who, alt-hough supportive at the start, become confused by the ongoing "drama" of the process and gradually drift away.

I never had to face regrowth of molar tissue, because in my year of waiting, my levels never rose. It was not necessary for me to have chemotherapy, so I cannot begin to describe or even imagine the endless nightmare that women with persistent GTD must go through. I remember one woman, one of the early members of my support group, who had been through multiple trials of chemotherapy regimens and had lost her hair and had to walk around attached to an intravenous line. She had a young daughter as well, and her little girl had to grow up seeing her mother sick, bald, tired, and attached to strange devices. Although this woman, like many others, went on to have a healthy pregnancy, her story broke my heart and has always stayed with me. Many of the stories in this book include treatment with chemotherapy, and I will leave it to those women who know best to describe that experience.

Supporting the Molar Patient

Friends and Family

It is during this crucial period that women need support and understanding most and are least likely to receive it. Support groups like mine and others have tried to fill this void. I have not come across any "real world" support groups for women with molar pregnancies in a very long time, and those for cho-riocarcinoma are unheard of, because the condition itself is so rare. Friends and family members often e-mail me with the same question: How can I help a loved one who has had a mo-lar pregnancy?

Family and friends should take their cues from the woman and her partner. Some couples prefer to keep their loss to them-selves, whereas others feel the need to talk. In many cases the woman wants to talk about it, but the partner does not. The best thing outsiders can do is offer support and a willing ear but not be persistent or ask for intimate details unless the woman, partner, or couple are willing to volunteer them. Most women with GTD seek answers more than anything else, so sharing this book and others like it, as well as websites that deal specifically with molar pregnancies can be helpful. Most of all, friends and family must be patient. Remember that this was not a "normal" miscarriage that the woman will just "get over." Every month for the foreseeable future she will be reminded of her loss and face renewed fear of regrowth and cancer. She won't be trying for another baby anytime soon, so don't ask things like "How's the babymaking going?" or "Are you trying to get pregnant again yet?" You'd be amazed how many people, even after being told about the waiting period and the risks, will nonetheless ask such insensitive and clueless questions.

Another important thing for supporters to remember is that although the woman is dealing with many things, she is primarily grieving. Her expectations of becoming a mother have been dashed. She has lost a child, and her life has been put on hold by a condition no one else has heard of—unless they too have been touched by it. She may desperately wish to have a baby, yet she cannot even try again for up to as long as a year. Women with GTD are left with the biggest question of all: Why me? In response, they often feel jealous of other women around them who are visibly pregnant. I can say from my own experience that when you've lost a child and are mourning that loss, it suddenly seems as though *every other woman on Earth* is pregnant except you. I remember glaring at random women on the street whose baby bumps were showing and thinking, "Why them and not me?" Coworkers and friends and family who are pregnant are even more likely targets for jealousy, because the grieving woman sees them and hears their happy stories on a regular basis. She knows it is wrong to be jealous, and in most cases she *wants* to be happy for the friend or relative who is pregnant, but the grief and jealousy can be overwhelming. Thus although the woman should not be *excluded* from baby-related events such as showers, her invitation should be offered with some sensitivity. If she declines an invitation, or does not seem to share in or listen to conversations about someone's new baby, this should be accepted gracefully. A woman who has lost a pregnancy should never be made to feel guilty or required to attend someone else's baby event, and the pregnant friend or family member should be willing to accept that the woman's absence or reticence is not intended as a personal offense.

Another difficult time for the woman with GTD is the arrival of her due date. As time passes after the diagnosis and the grief and shock wear off, things may return to normal. However, the woman has not forgotten that she was "supposed to be pregnant." Most women, on learning they are pregnant, immediately try to determine their due date. Mine was December 5, 2001; after all this time I still remember it, and when it comes, I think of my loss for a moment or two, even now. The woman's friends and family can best help by remembering that date as well, at least in that first year, and doing what they can to take the woman's mind off her loss. She may well become depressed and moody, morose, or tearful. She may shut herself off from others during that time. Help her get out of the house. Don't leave her to mourn alone.

Doctors and Other Medical Personnel

I have said that women share a common complaint about the way they are treated by their medical practitioners after a molar pregnancy diagnosis. Before I go any further, let me say this: Although I have heard many horror stories, I have also heard wonderful stories about truly caring and supportive physicians and nurses. Not everyone has a bad experience. However, there is a common feeling among most of the women I've corresponded with that their doctors, especially their primary care physicians and gynecologists, are too inexperienced, uninformed, or regimented in their approach to molar pregnancies. The rare occurrence of GTD makes it something few doctors ever treat, and thus the "standard approach" —i.e., the one they learned in medical school years ago or found online or in a textbook after a quick search, an approach that is quickly becoming outdated—is the only approach they can accept. Doctors generally don't like to be told they are wrong, and many are affronted by patients who bring in research or argue against "standard" treatment. Yet many of the women in my groups have done just that. When faced with physicians who are unwilling to accept another approach or another line of thought, these women often take their care into their own hands, cutting short their monitoring periods to conceive again or going "doctor shopping" to find a physician more willing to negotiate. I have argued against this practice many times in my support groups, urging women to follow their doctors' orders, but for the doctor–patient relationship to work, the doctor has to meet the patient halfway.

If changes to the treatment regimen are not appropriate, the doctor should be forthcoming about the reasons and the evidence that support his or her stance. There are too many emotions involved in this situation for a doctor to take a position based on the "I know best, that's why" theory. Communication and trust between the woman and her doctor are the key elements to adherence and understanding on both sides. It is time consuming (and unlikely) for doctors who rarely, if ever, treat a woman with GTD to go online or rummage through back issues of medical journals to find the latest research, particularly when there is a "standard approach" available. A patient who does her own research and brings it in to the doctor, however, has eliminated some of the legwork and offered an opportunity for further discussion, education, and experience. This kind of proactive involvement in treatment should be welcomed, not discouraged or ignored. Most of all, the woman should not be condescended to, patted on the head like a trained dog, or otherwise disrespected for her efforts. She is trying to come to terms with a situation beyond her control. Encourage, support, and be proactive along with her.

Another issue that physicians need to address when they encounter a patient with a molar pregnancy is the education of their staff and related medical personnel about the diagnosis. Charts should be clearly marked so that nurses or laboratory technicians do not mistake the woman as a "prenatal" case and offer her congratulations and a cup to pee in. A staff meeting should be held or a memo issued to staff members that describes molar pregnancy and its attendant risks. The patient should not be subjected to insensitive, uninformed, or impertinent questions. When the woman calls in for her laboratory results each month or receives a call from the office about the results, the staff member receiving or making the call should remember that the woman is waiting to hear if she might have to have chemotherapy for a regrowth or cancer. Messages and conversations should be sensitive and to the point. Friendly chatter can follow if the news is good. I had a wonderful nurse I spoke to each month at my medical center when my results came in, and having the same person on the line each time became a comfort to me, because I knew she understood what I was going through and was helping me through it one month at a time. She was my lifeline in the office, and when I encountered other staff who were clueless or insensitive, she would step in for me and clear everything up. When I was cleared to conceive again, she cheered for me and we hugged. When I came in pregnant four months later, she was ecstatic. Confidentiality issues may make some of these recommendations impractical, but steps nonetheless should be taken to ensure these women do not feel ignored, rejected, or misunderstood when visiting their physician.

In summary, the people around a woman with GTD—whether they be friends, family, or medical personnel entrusted with her care—need to understand the wide range of emotions she is feeling and her unique needs during this time. They need to be sensitive to her loss, her grief, and her fears. They need to be patient as she struggles with her diagnosis, educates herself about her condition, and carries on through the lengthy period of monitoring and recovery. If she requires chemotherapy, supporters should take the time to learn the side effects of the treatment and offer assistance with household tasks or other responsibilities when she is too tired or sick to take care of them herself. Supporters and physicians should remember that the partner in the couple has experienced a loss as well and is living in a state of fear for the woman's health, and they should offer whatever help or comfort the partner will accept. Physicians, particularly those with little practical experience with molar pregnancies, should be open minded and willing to go the extra mile in researching the condition when the woman seeks additional information or asks for changes in the treatment regimen. Finally, medical staff should be given the opportunity to learn more about the condition and be trained to handle any women who have had a miscarriage—regardless of cause!—with sensitivity and care.

A Word About Science Versus Emotion

Most women, when diagnosed with a molar pregnancy, will do just as I did: they will go online and look for more information. There is a lot more information and support out there today than there was in 2001, when most of what I found was technical jargon. Nonetheless, in all likelihood, these women will find at least one article or blog post or comment stating unequivocally that there is "no fetus" in a molar pregnancy, and therefore it is *not a real pregnancy.*

It is not my goal or even my desire to enter into a debate about what constitutes a fetus, baby, or child. However, the statement that "there is no baby" in a molar pregnancy has caused a great deal of confusion and distress to me and to many of the women I have heard from during the years. Over time, I have found that women with molar pregnancies tend to split into groups with regard to how they choose to respond to this scientific observation. At one end of the spectrum are women who choose to embrace the science. Believing that there was no baby and no pregnancy to begin with offers them a way of avoiding grief for a life lost and a means of detaching any "motherly" emotions from the situation. At the other end of the spectrum are women who have not only rejected the science but have gone so far as to name their lost child and/or bury the molar tissue, even holding services or creating memorials to the child. In the middle are most women, those who simply don't know what to believe in and are left with an empty feeling that neither science nor faith can fully satisfy.

I can't offer a solution or a definitive answer as to what to believe in. I am not a particularly religious person, but I am also not a strict devotée of science. In my personal experience, when I took that pregnancy test in 2001 and it came back positive, I was pregnant. No one will ever convince me otherwise. In my heart and in my mind I bonded with the child I thought was growing inside me. I planned a future for my baby. I designed a nursery and shared my good news with my family and friends. For four short weeks I was a mother, and although I never saw or felt a baby, to me that child existed, however briefly. I have accepted, with the passage of time and through my work on the MyMolarPregnancy.com website, that there never was an actual physical life growing inside me. But there was the *spirit* of a child, and the *hope* and *dream* of a child, and that is the reality I choose to live with. Whatever reality you choose to believe in, let it be the one that brings you the most comfort and the least pain.

Reference

Johnson T, Schwartz M: *Gestational Trophoblastic Neoplasia: A Guide for Women Dealing With Tumors of the Placenta, such as Choriocarcinoma, Molar Pregnancy, and Other Forms of GTN.* Victoria, BC, Canada, Trafford Publishing, 2007

Amber

Molar pregnancy. Yes, I had read the term in parenting books, but I knew it was rare and probably would not happen to me.

But it did. Twice.

Let me back up a bit. We had at the time two amazing kids, L and B. L was three and a half years old, and B was almost two years old. I became pregnant without really trying that third time, and I'm not sure when it happened, but I pegged it around March 17, 2009. I had suspicions and took a test in the bathroom at Wal-Mart. In the dark stall I thought I saw a faint line. I returned home and told my husband, but he thought it was wrong, so I had him buy another test a few days later. The line that appears that time was unmistakable—we were expecting baby number three! I was excited; I had always dreamed of having three children. My husband was still in shock. A few days later I had some spotting, but I am blood type O negative and would need a shot of WinRho anyway, so I waited to see the doctor. It was the Saturday before Easter, and I didn't want to ruin my kids' weekend. On the following Monday I went to a local emergency room and waited. My nurse was very kind. She drew blood, and the doctor performed an ultrasound. I was only five weeks along, so nothing could be seen aside from the sac. I was given the shot and sent on my way. By Friday night I was already worrying about having three kids and a small car, so we bought a minivan. We began thinking of names, and I settled on Cameron Riley, because both of my other kids had seven letters in their first names. It was perfect!

Saturday morning I woke and went to the bathroom as usual. I got up to see blood and pieces of tissue in the toilet. I was alarmed, but I thought it was my Crohn's disease misbehaving. Still, I thought I should revisit the emergency room just to be sure. My husband dropped me off and took the kids to their gymnastics and swimming with the help of a friend. In the hospital I was assigned a distant room where I sat alone, freezing, and crying. I had my iPod with me and listened to it to pass the time. I started cramping, and I knew something was wrong, but a second round of blood work and another ultrasound showed no problems. I was told to return the next morning for an ultrasound at ten o'clock.

I went home and waited, still unsure about what was happening. I returned to the hospital alone again the next day. The ultrasound started half an hour late. The technician asked how far along I was, because he could see a sac but no fetal pole nor heartbeat, which should have been visible at seven weeks. I was sent to their family waiting room to await a bed. In shock, I called my husband and told him the news. The rest of the conversation was a blur. Once I was assigned a bed a doctor came in and concurred that the pregnancy was gone. He told me miscarriages are common, and one-quarter of all pregnancies end in miscarriage. As I was leaving, I encountered the nurse from Monday's tests, and she showed me that my hCG level had risen from the previous visit's results. Perhaps that foreshadowed things to come.

I drove home dazed and teary. I had had a miscarriage. The only person I knew who had had one before me was my mother-in-law, thirty-plus years earlier. No help there. I spoke with a friend, ate lunch, and went to bed. Days passed, and I was zombie-like. I had no way of knowing the hard times were yet to come.

The next week was our son's second birthday. During his party my mother-in-law asked the unthinkable: "Time for another?" She didn't know that anything had happened. My friends covered for me and distracted her to prevent a blowout occurring. I took our son in for his two-year checkup, and the doctor gave me a blood work prescription to check my beta hCG level. She advised that I wait until April 30, which I did. A week afterward she called and kept saying, "I'm puzzled." About what? I thought. You're the doctor! She informed me my hCG level had risen and wanted me in as soon as possible for an ultrasound. Problem was, I was home alone with the kids, my husband was at work with the van, and hospital policy forbade kids coming in with a mother alone. After some arranging my in-laws arrived, and my mother-in-law stayed with the kids while my father-in-law drove me to the doctor.

They took me in for another ultrasound. The technician confirmed that yes, I had miscarried, but that I would need to talk to the doctors on call. Half an hour passed, and I was placed in another room. My husband had arrived but was out somewhere with my father-in-law waiting for me. To this day I wish he had been with me. The doctor and student arrived and dropped the news on me. I think they gave me a quick rundown, but must admit I was shell shocked and only remember "Blah, blah, blah, molar pregnancy, rare, cancer," and so on. I came in believing I had had a miscarriage but was leaving with a tumor inside of me? They did an internal ultrasound and told me I would need to have my D&C in two days. The department that would handle it was closed and would not be able to do it sooner. Then they said, "We have no pamphlets [about molar pregnancy]; go home and Google." They actually told me to turn to the Internet!

At some point I found my husband, and we left. The next day, Thursday, was a blur. I was still in a fog and so confused; I searched Google and started telling some friends about what had happened, but they didn't know what to say. I also nursed my two-year-old for the last time that day, a bittersweet memory in so many ways.

My appointment for the D&C was on Friday, May 8, 2009, which was also my husband's day off. My own gynecologist was not there but after the necessary blood draws, weight/height measurements, and blood pressure test another doctor came in and went over everything with me. She asked if I wanted to be totally unconscious for the procedure, and after speaking with a friend about it I said yes. I went back to the preoperative waiting area, and eventually they came to get me. I was terrified, afraid I would not wake up from this minor procedure. I remember lying on the table with my legs in the ugly black stirrups and having my intravenous line put in, but I don't remember much after that until I woke in recovery. I remember they could not find my husband to come and get me. They claimed they had called his cellphone, and later he claimed he never received a call. After an hour he finally arrived. I remember the drive home; it was a bright, sunny, warm day. When we arrived home I stopped to see my kids for a moment and then crashed into bed.

Less than twenty-four hours later my husband was called into work. His boss could not care less that I had to have someone with me for the first twenty-four hours because of the medication I'd been given. That's the military for you!

The next day was Mother's Day, and it was brutal. I was not feeling myself; I was broken and hurt and just wanted to stay in bed, but my husband insisted it was his mom's day as well and we should see her. At the same time a close friendship ended badly, and I felt very alone. I had no other mom friends I could turn to. Instead I slept a lot and cried myself to sleep. When I finally reached out for help I was put in touch with a spiritual care leader at the hospital who was also my husband's unit padre. Due to some past issues we had had with him, he passed my case along to a coworker, Colleen. She and I spoke for two hours, not about the loss of the baby but of my friendship as well. She mentioned grief counseling in a group setting, and I thought it would help. My husband and I started group counseling with two other couples. They had had losses much farther along than ours and although they were great people, I felt we did not belong there.

In the weeks that passed, I went through the motions but couldn't get past my loss. My heart felt raw. At one point our eldest said, "Here, Mommy. You take Lexie [her stuffed animal]. She can be your baby." This only made me cry more. My hormones were crazy. Nothing was concrete yet because we were still waiting for pathology results to confirm the molar. My post-D&C bleeding lasted for two months, and it was heavy and awful. I filled super-absorbency tampons every hour. I called the hospital only to be told that it was normal and that I was not to come in.

I turned to the Internet and tried to reason and figure out why this happened. The only thing I learned was that there was no reason. The information I found was all over the place. One page said one thing, whereas another said something else.

This loss hit me much harder than it did my husband. I was the one going through weekly blood draws. I was even asked at one point how far along I was, and when I explained about our loss the technician said, "Oh, we saw a molar pregnancy picture from the seventies in a medical text book, it had hair and teeth."

Not helpful.

Days passed and became weeks, and I was still having weekly blood draws. Fortunately the woman who managed all the molar pregnancy monitoring was great about calling each week after she got the results. At some point two months after my D&C I had to track down the gynecologist to get the official diagnosis because no one had called me. She confirmed that it had been a complete molar pregnancy but dismissed my worries about cancer, saying, "That only happens in underdeveloped countries." Wrong! I was lucky that I never developed cancer, but to dismiss me in that way was not cool.

I don't recall my exact hCG levels, but at some point after three weeks of negative results (considered a level of 3 or less here) I switched to monthly. Yay! Yet when I switched to monthly draws I still relived everything twice a month, once during the blood draw and once when my period arrived. Nature mocked me, never letting them happen the same time. It was always every two weeks, either a draw or a period.

That summer, knowing I was not allowed to get pregnant, I started medication for back pain that had troubled me since our eldest's birth. One made me loopy and wired for sound, keeping me up until four in the morning. At this point I was both mom and dad, because summer training had called my husband away. My doctor switched me to Lyrica, which made me gain weight. I was unhappy and still upset over our loss. I hurt and had no support and was running on empty.

Our tenth wedding anniversary approached, and my husband kept asking what I wanted to do. I spotted a Disney sign, and that was the answer! I'm a Disney freak. That trip helped a lot. Christmas came and passed. In January I was given the six-month all-clear but was told it would be better to wait until twelve months had passed. It was a weird time. We wanted another child and were cleared to try for it, but I was terrified it would happen all over again. We waited another six months. When July came, my last call with my nurse was bittersweet: She was lovely but I never wanted to have to call her again.

Time passed, and soon it was autumn 2010. Our eldest started school. I was friends with some other women who had had losses, but I still did not feel I fit in. I turned to Facebook and found molar pregnancy groups that were becoming more active. Was this a good thing? Yes, but it was sad that more women were dealing with this.

In May 2011 I took the kids and a friend to Disney on my own. It was not the best trip. My daughter landed in the emergency room with a double ear infection, my Crohn's disease decided in the emergency room it would be a good time to flare, and my husband and I nearly broke up. We flew home on Mother's Day and had dinner out. That night we made up and had sex. I was not on any birth control and we didn't use protection. Then just as June was arriving I had a strong suspicion I was pregnant again. I left the house early in the morning and bought a test, and sure enough, it was positive! Eek!

The next weekend was a guided camping event that had us walking all over downtown. During the event, I started to bleed—not a lot, but the cramps and bleeding hurt, and it worried me. Shortly afterward I saw the doctor for another WinRho shot and an ultrasound. We saw the heartbeat and the technician assured us the brown blood I had had was just old blood. We moved onward. Surely it couldn't be happening again. It was too rare.

I went in for my first gynecology appointment and explained I had been bleeding. I was put in a room for another ultrasound. After looking at the screen, the doctor said, "Well, it's an old machine, so I can't see much." She printed a picture and left. Half an hour later, she and her supervising doctor came in. He told me they were pretty sure I had miscarried again. Again I was alone with this news. Hubby was en route from work five minutes down the road. He couldn't believe it. When he arrived and found me the doctor told us they wanted more blood work and another ultrasound in two days. I made it out of the room and down the hall to the huge waiting room before I let out a sob. From there I could not stop crying. Not again, not another loss! Was this it for us? We would only have the two children we had now? At home I went to bed, where I prayed and cried.

Friday morning my husband he dropped me off for my tests and left to take our daughter to summer camp and our son to his parents. I had the blood drawn and went to the early pregnancy complications clinic. They put me in a room and when the doctor came in I had to explain why I was there and my while history. He knew little and joked that I should be documenting it because I knew it better than he did. My room was next to the staff area, and I overheard them say that I was in for an abortion and the words *molar pregnancy*. It broke my heart. I know the term *abortion* is just a medical term, but in my heart and head that was not a word I wanted to hear.

Hubby finally returned, and we were sent down to ultrasound again. The technician was sweet to us, but there was no heartbeat on the monitor. She confirmed the worst and gave us her sympathies and left us with the Kleenex box. "Take as long as you need," she told us. We left and I sobbed all the way upstairs again. I had been told I would be having the D&C that day, but they could not fit me in. Another doctor and student came in to do the internal exam and were thrown by the fact that we had seen the heartbeat this time but still were thinking another molar. My uterus felt large for how far along I was supposed to be. They gave me a choice: I could let it go, take pills, or have a D&C. With a vow renewal in Jamaica set for two weeks later I elected for the D&C.

I left the hospital with information about molar pregnancy and miscarriage loss. I called my nurse from the previous molar pregnancy immediately, and she called me back and talked me down a bit. At some point the hospital called to schedule Monday's surgery. That weekend I stupidly watched *Marley and Me* and bawled when Jenny lost the baby. That night my husband and I made love, and it was very touching. It was the release we needed. On Monday morning I arrived at the hospital and went through all the preoperative things I had gone through already two years ago. It was eerie. This time my own gynecologist performed the surgery. She recommended that I not be knocked out, but I think at some point I was out anyway. I wish I had asked to see what was left of the baby; I waited too long and did not ask until I was already in recovery.

We returned home and I saw tiger lilies growing in our yard. I named this baby Lily. I said "Hi" to the kids, then went to bed and slept. My recovery was much better this time, with mild spotting for only three or four days. We left for Jamaica, and although I had a bit more spotting while we were there, it was nothing compared with what I'd had two years prior. We renewed our vows, drank, and had fun, and for the most part I didn't dwell. On the last day I did worry a bit and wonder about the usual "What ifs."

Friday, July 29, my gynecologist called with the results: partial molar pregnancy. I was angry. Not again! This is insane! She told me what I needed to do, which of course I already knew being the old pro. I contacted my nurse again, and she said, "Okay, let's get on it." The only bright side was a shorter wait this time. I did weekly testing into September. Two weeks of blood work went missing when the hospital lost the vials while I was there for iron infusions. When my nurse called and said my level was 5 (remember my nurse wanted 3 or lower), I was fit to be tied. I cried. I had only one week left, but that was one more week away from a baby. One week doesn't seem like a long time, but after two losses and a lot of waiting, it felt like a knife to the heart.

In October I went off the pill again, and in November I was given the all-clear to conceive. I knew my body, and I knew when I was ovulating. Yet when we became pregnant the first week of December we find out because my nurse called on December 20 with slight alarm in her voice. My level had risen!

I assured her it was possible I was pregnant, but she wanted blood work drawn as quickly as possible. However, we were leaving for Disney the next morning. While we were there I picked up a stomach bug from my daughter and was miserable into the new year. On New Year's Eve I was in the shower and passed clots. I freaked but knew nothing could be done, so I stayed in the room. When we came home I went to see my doctor immediately. She was convinced it was a miscarriage and sent me for blood and another WinRho shot.

Three and a half hours later she called me with terrible news: "Amber, your level is 67,000. It's a third molar." I told her, "I'm done, I want a hysterectomy. No way can you avoid cancer three times." She answered that it was probably a good idea. I went to the Internet. My level was in the middle range for a pregnancy of six to seven weeks. I cried, I prayed, I worried.

Two days later I had another ultrasound. It was January and freezing. The technician was the same one we had had for the first ultrasound with molar number two. We were fully expecting this one to end badly as well. My husband and I looked at the screen and saw it at the same time: a heartbeat! I squeezed his hand. The technician saw it as well and calculated the estimated delivery date as August 29, 2012. It was a sign! That was the same date as our daughter's seventh birthday! This one was a keeper.

Two more ultrasounds had to be scheduled before I could be given the all-clear to announce our pregnancy. The next one appointment was slated for February 12. How would I not go insane for five weeks? I made it, and although my husband had to go to Virginia that morning, he got good news before he left: the baby was still there and in great shape. Another ultrasound the next week, and then I was finally fourteen weeks and they told me I could share the news. I have never seen my Facebook account blow up so fast!

The pregnancy was not without its bumps, and I had ten or eleven ultrasounds along the way. The doctors watched me like hawks. However, Natalie Rebecca Hope arrived on August 30 at 2:59 p.m. Her delivery was medication free, but not because I planned it that way! She was jaundiced and there was some concern that her hip clicked oddly, but it was nothing. We say she's a born trouble maker who started in the womb! As I write this she is nearly ten months old and a busy girl. She is a boatload of trouble but truly a welcome and longed-for addition to the family. She completes us.

I have no inspiring words of wisdom that other molar pregnancy ladies haven't heard before. However, here is my advice: grieve. You have every right to. Celebrate your baby how you want him or her to be remembered. You lost a baby and your dreams for the future. That pain will never leave entirely but will diminish. You will get through this. I promise. It does not feel like that now, but you *will* get through it, and you will be stronger in the end. If you are able to have a child you will love him or her an insane amount that your heart did not think possible. If you are unable to have another baby, I promise it will be alright in time. Grieve. This is a big loss to let go and realize. You need time to heal as well.

For those just starting their molar journey, I'm sorry you're here. No one needs to endure this. It hurts. It sucks. We lose control of everything. We don't fit into the normal miscarriage groups, but we had a loss too. If you need help, ask for it. Do not suffer alone. The fear of cancer and the "what if" questions while you wait for your results each week are nerve wracking. This disease plays with your emotions, your heart, and your mind. This too will pass.

I look back at my two molar pregnancies and say "Wow, I went through that twice? What on Earth?" (Those aren't the words I would really use, but I have to keep it clean!) It seems a small blip now, and yet certain aspects are so fresh in my mind. You will hear that it wasn't meant to be, that God had other plans, etc., none of which seem be helpful to you. Just know deep down that people don't say these things to be hurtful. They are sad for your loss and pain and do not know how else to reach out.

Miscarriage in general is a taboo subject. Throw in the science of a molar pregnancy and you have people heading for the hills. You and those around you will have questions:

- What do you mean a pregnancy can cause cancer?
- Did *you* do anything to cause this?
- Will you have another mole?
- What *is* a molar pregnancy?

You will also be faced with comments that hurt or may even seem mean, although they may in fact be meant to help or support you:

- It wasn't a baby.
- Be thankful you lost it early, before you were attached.
- It's been months, get over it.

No one has the right to tell you to get over it or that it was never a baby. It was *your* baby (or not, depending on how you *want* to see it), and your dream for the future. I'm sending hugs to you all. This is not an easy road, but you will survive it and be stronger for it. It is amazing, the strength we have as women!

Amy

My husband and I got married in October 2008. We knew we wanted to have kids right away. We waited a few months since we had just married, but by February 2009 we were ready to start trying. On March 6, 2009, I found out I was pregnant. Wow! I did not think it would be that easy! My husband and I were thrilled. Little did I know what we were in for.

I had my first appointment with the obstetrician later that week for what they called "a confirmation" appointment. Basically, the office performed another pregnancy test, congratulated me, and scheduled me for an ultrasound three weeks later, when I would be seven weeks pregnant.

About a week after my confirmation appointment, I started spotting red blood. I called the doctor right away, and they told me not to worry and that that can happen in early pregnancy, but if it got worse to call them back. At that point, I was not really worried because I still felt terrible, which I figured was a good sign, and the spotting stopped. A few days later, it started again and continued right up to that first ultrasound. By that point, I was a little worried.

I don't remember much about that first ultrasound, other than the technician saying that the baby was measuring small and that the heartbeat was a little low. I asked what the heartbeat was, and she said seventy-three beats per minute. I had read enough about fetal ultrasounds to know seventy-three at seven weeks pregnant was really bad. She then asked us to wait in the hall, because the doctor wanted to talk to us. I sat there feeling as though I might vomit. It didn't help that while we sat there another couple walked by with both their parents, all of them ecstatic because they were about to find out if they were having a boy or girl. A few minutes later, the doctor called us back to a room. I will never forget her; she was so kind. She explained that the ultrasound did not look good and that we should come back the following Monday (it was Friday) because we would probably know what was going on by then. She then let us ask questions. I think that was the longest weekend of my life.

When we returned on Monday, the ultrasound results confirmed what we already knew was coming: I had had a miscarriage, but my body was not yet ready to let go of the pregnancy. The doctor told us I could either wait for my body to miscarry on its own or have a D&C. I opted for a D&C because I was not up for just waiting for things to happen. The doctor scheduled the procedure for that Thursday. I think I spent those next three days continually crying.

I went in for surgery on April 8, 2009. I was a complete mess. My preoperative nurse was amazing. She told me she was sorry we were meeting under those circumstances and explained that she had had four miscarriages, so she knew what I was going through. My husband was not allowed back to wait with me before the surgery, but she made me feel much less alone. Then she asked me if I wanted a "cocktail," or some drugs to take the edge off. That made me laugh a bit and I answered, "Yes, please!" The next thing I remember was waking up in recovery. The weird thing is that when I woke up, I felt physically better. I shook it off and just thought it was normal. Knowing what I now know about molars, I should have clued in that this was anything but a "normal" miscarriage.

After the surgery, we were told everything went well, that I would probably bleed for a week to ten days, and that I should return in two weeks to make sure everything was okay. After the D&C I had a hard time holding myself together. I cried all the time. I also read everything online that I could about miscarriage and began to wonder if I was ever going to be able to have kids. I also became worried because my bleeding didn't seem to be stopping and was really heavy. I called the doctor and she told me not to worry about it.

Going to the obstetrician's office for my follow-up appointment two weeks later was extremely difficult. It was so hard to walk into a room full of happy pregnant women. I broke down when they asked me to give them a urine sample and yelled at the receptionist that it wasn't necessary because I wasn't pregnant anymore. Then the doctor called me back. I remember thinking that she had such a serious look on her face. I knew I wasn't the most fun appointment of the day, but I didn't understand her expression. Then she started explaining that I had had a partial molar pregnancy. When I told her I had never heard of a molar pregnancy, she explained that there were two types of moles, complete and partial, and that I had had the less serious of the two. She then took a long time explaining that moles can, in certain circumstances, cause cancer because the molar tissue may grow back.

I think I stopped listening when she said the word *cancer*. In my case, she said the likelihood of cancer was only about five percent, but that I could not get pregnant for six months because they needed to monitor me to make sure the mole did not come back. If it did, I was going to need a low-dose chemotherapy called methotrexate. In the meantime, I had to have my hCG hormone monitored every two weeks because that was the only way to know if the mole was growing back. She then asked if I had any questions. I think I just stared at her blankly. I then had my hCG level checked. The doctor had told me that nonpregnant women have an hCG level of less than 2. Mine was 494, which, if I had actually been pregnant, would have put me at five weeks. I found that ironic because I was two weeks post D&C.

I learned over the next few weeks that the hCG hormone drops very slowly in people who have had moles. Two weeks later mine was 44. Two weeks after that, it was 21. Then it was 11. At that point the bleeding finally stopped. However, about a week later I woke in the middle of the night covered in blood. I panicked and was convinced the mole had returned. I placed an emergency call to my doctor. She told me to come in first thing in the morning. When I arrived, she ordered an ultra-sound to see if there was anything left in my uterus. They were able to see a small piece of retained pregnancy tissue, which the doctor removed in the office. She said that would probably take care of the problem, but she wanted to check my hCG level anyway to make sure they did not go up. My level was at 8, so it was still dropping. That was such a relief. Two weeks later it was at 5. I was frustrated that it was starting to drop so slowly, but she told me not to worry and that levels dropped more slowly the closer you got to zero. By early June, my hCG level was finally less than 2.

After my level finally reached normal, I really fell apart. While I was waiting I had been okay because I had my health to worry about, but once that was out of the way, depression set in. I cried all the time and could not leave my house without losing it completely. I couldn't handle being around my friends or anyone who knew what had happened. It also didn't help that my family was less than understanding. They thought I should have just gotten "over it." As if things are always that simple. Thank goodness for my husband. He was my rock and let me do whatever I needed, which was mostly cry. If I wasn't crying, I was doing home improvement projects to keep my mind off things. Those were probably the worst few months of my life.

At the end of June 2009, I went to my doctor for my monthly blood draw to make sure my hCG level was still at zero. I told her about some research I had run across by Dr.

Goldstein, who is *the* molar expert in the United States, that said that if the hCG level dropped in someone who had had a partial molar pregnancy within seven weeks, the waiting period only needed to be three months and not six months. She reviewed the research and agreed I fit into that category, so she dropped my waiting period to three months, or August 2009. I was ecstatic, because it was already late June, so I only had to wait one month more before we could try to get pregnant again.

At the end of August 2009, I had some weird bleeding that started and stopped within a few hours about a week before my period was due. It was really upsetting to me because I was starting to feel like my body would never be "normal" again. A few days later, I realized my period was late, despite the bleeding. I realized that the bleeding may have been implantation bleeding, but I waited a few days before taking a pregnancy test. It was positive. I would like to say I was excited to be pregnant again, but I wasn't. I was freaked out. I called my doctor immediately. She told me to come in to have my hCG level checked. My level was 1,100. Four days later, it was 10,000, so my hCG was doubling as it should for where I was in the pregnancy.

Three weeks later, the seven-week ultrasound looked perfect. Everyone in my doctor's office congratulated me, but I still could not relax. I kept thinking something was going to go wrong. It didn't help that I had spotting every week during the first trimester. My doctor was amazing; she let me come in for an ultrasound nearly every week during that time to reassure me everything was okay. After the spotting stopped and I had made it through the first trimester, I still had a hard time believing everything was going to be okay. I drove my husband crazy with my obsessive worrying, but everything worked out just fine.

On April 28, 2010, I gave birth by cesarean section to an eight-pound, four-ounce baby girl. She was perfect and so completely worth the wait. I really cannot imagine not having her. After twenty-two months and two "normal" miscarriages, her sister joined us on February 28, 2012. As I type this story now, we are nine weeks away from completing our family in August 2013 when our third little girl will arrive.

When my husband and I set out on our journey to start a family, we never knew things would take the twists and turns that they did. There was a time that I really thought that I would never have the family that I had always wanted. Luckily, that didn't happen and everything worked out, as it most often does. As hard as it was to go through the molar pregnancy and everything that went with it, I would do it again in a heartbeat because I cannot imagine life without my kids. They are perfect (to me anyway), and I appreciate them so much more because of how hard I had to work to have them. I am extremely lucky to have the family that I do and I wouldn't change it for the world.

Becky

I heard my husband come home for breakfast after his required morning physical training. I couldn't wait to tell him what I had just learned—we were pregnant! Just three weeks earlier our three daughters and I had welcomed him home from a twelve-month deployment with the U.S. Army to Iraq. Apparently we conceived eight days after his return.

I was thrilled. We had wanted another child for a long time, but army life kept getting in the way. Before this year-long deployment, we had moved from one duty station to another; before that, he had been deployed for fifteen months, also to Iraq. Our youngest daughter was now four and a half years old, so there would be a big age gap between her and her new sibling. I wasn't getting any younger either. I was one month away from turning thirty-five years old, when the obstetric clinics kindly begin to refer to you as "AMA"— advanced maternal age. I felt old to be expecting another child, for some reason, but I strongly desired to have at least one, possibly two more children.

I sat next to my husband at the table. "We're going to need that new minivan sooner than we thought," I told him. He half-choked on his cereal, and then looked at me with surprise.

"That was quick," he said. "Wow. Okay."

"Yep, I should be due December fourth. Are you excited?"

"Yeah." [Pause.] "That'll mean we'll have to request that the army not move us until at least next year in the summer then." Men. They're always thinking of logistics.

My parents were coming in a few days for a visit, but we decided not to tell them until after I'd had my first appointment. I hadn't scheduled an appointment yet, but I expected would get around to it after their visit. It was torturous having this secret, feeling the beginnings of first-trimester symptoms while cooking and entertaining my parents. I was really tired. I wasn't nauseous, really, but I definitely felt bloated. I made it through their entire visit without spilling the beans, but it was just a few days later that I felt the need to tell our children. Being kids, though, they would likely not be able to keep a secret from our community, so I figured I'd better call our parents and make the announcement first. My parents were thrilled. His parents were caught off guard (I assume because of my age). Over the next several days I enjoyed breaking the news to friends. I was so excited. Finally, we would have our fourth child! I scheduled my appointment with the OB/GYN clinic at our local army hospital.

That first visit was only a consultation, a chance to give them my medical history and the date of my last menstrual period and to get information from them about the clinic. They scheduled me to see one of their midwives for my first appointment on Wednesday, May 18. I would be eleven and a half weeks along by then, because I'd waited awhile to call and start the whole process and obstetric clinics at army hospitals are quite busy. It could not come soon enough.

We went to my appointment mostly anticipating hearing the heartbeat. Our older children were at school, and our youngest was with a friend. The midwife seemed great, and I was looking forward to working with her over the coming months. She started right away with a portable ultrasound that would also pick up sound. I turned my head to the screen and cocked my ears for that familiar sound, which I hadn't heard in a few years. She seemed to be having some trouble locating where the baby was. I didn't recognize what was on the screen, but then, ultra-sounds are confusing to those without a trained eye.

After a couple of minutes, she said, "Let me go get the doctor to confirm what I'm seeing." That did not sound good. Perhaps there were twins? I waited. The doctor came in and introduced himself and quickly took over the ultrasound. It wasn't long before he spoke.

"I'm sorry, but this is not a viable pregnancy." What in the world did that mean? He explained: "I think what we're seeing here is a molar pregnancy. There is no baby. It's just a mass of tissue. We need to send you down to radiology to confirm some things, and then I'd like you to come back to my office and I'll explain more about what's going on."

I looked at my husband with confusion, fear, and disappointment. As I went down to radiology for a more thorough ultrasound, I already knew I wasn't going to have a baby in December, but I was still very confused as to *why*. I had already had three healthy pregnancies that went full term with few to no complications. Was it my age? This was not a normal miscarriage. It was all so strange.

I finished with the ultrasound, and then we met with the doctor, who looked over the radiology report and confirmed his diagnosis. He was extremely helpful and caring. He explained the two types of molar pregnancy and said that in my case, a complete mole, what likely happened was that my egg had had no genetic information. When it was fertilized, then, it only had one set of chromosomes and thus not enough information to produce a baby. Therefore, it simply produced a mass of tissue, "like a placenta gone wild," he said.

He went on to explain that I would need to have a D&C, which I had never heard of, so he described that as well and explained why I would need to have my hCG level tested regularly until it went down to zero. He was very thorough, and I am so thankful for his being well informed and explaining it so well to us. My D&C was then scheduled for that Friday, with preoperative registration set for the day before. This was not at all what I had expected from this day.

Looking back, I remember the midwife measuring the height of my fundus, and from that result she had thought I was farther along than I had stated. I had had neither spotting nor any other indicators that something was wrong. I remember having had a huge craving for meat, especially red meat. I also remember feeling as though my baby was a more noticeable presence in my belly much earlier in the pregnancy this time. Things definitely seemed to be expanding inside of me more rapidly. In hindsight, it did feel more like a "mass" than a normal pregnancy, as though there were a grapefruit or softball inside. Of course, not having been pregnant for a few years, I didn't trust my memories of my previous first trimesters or how things had felt. My early showing could be explained by the fact that this was my fourth pregnancy. I also remember having lots of heartburn.

My friend had picked up our older daughters from school, so we went to her house to get the kids. I cried as I explained to her, "There is no baby," and explained what I had learned about molar pregnancies. She was supportive and caring, even offering to provide us with meals, but I didn't feel I needed meals. What I really needed was reassurance and information about what to expect from this D&C procedure. I was nervous and concerned about that.

I spent that evening searching and reading about molar pregnancies. I appreciated the simple explanation given by WebMD, and I was grateful to find Facebook support groups where I could interact with others who had gone through the same thing. It was so strange, placing myself in this group of women experiencing this rare condition I had never heard of before.

As an army wife, I have learned to take hardships head-on and plow through them to the best of my ability. I focus on providing what is needed for my family and myself. I'm sure this affected how I dealt with this loss. My immediate focus was not on having lost a baby. "There is no baby," the doctor had said. So I didn't have any little person to care for, only myself. My focus was my own health and how I would face the D&C. After that, I reasoned, I would be able to grieve the loss.

The day I went for preoperative registration, the nurse gave me literature on miscarriages, even though she knew I was in a special situation. It included information about how this type of loss may affect extended family, and I immediately thought of my mother. I'd called her the day we found out about the molar pregnancy and told her what I knew. Only a few short weeks earlier we'd announced the joyful news of our pregnancy, and she had already started sewing baby bibs. This news hit her hard. She offered to tell my siblings and grandparents, which I accepted; I did not feel like explaining this unique thing to so many people right then. My sister later told me that my older brother also took it hard, and I received a rare phone call from him during that time to express his sympathy. I guess he felt protective toward me, his younger sister.

I was nervous going in for the D&C, but once the intravenous line started administering the anesthetic, I drifted off quickly. The next thing I remember was someone talking to me.

"Becky, you can wake up now. We're all done, and we're taking you to the recovery room."

My stretcher was wheeled down a hall into a room, and I was helped to the hospital bed while a nurse watched my vitals and asked how I felt. My legs were shaking, a symptom of the anesthetic. I was also very cold. Eventually those symptoms faded away, and soon I sat up with the nurse's help. My husband came into the room, and shortly afterward I was able to dress. Then I was wheeled to the entrance so my husband could take me home.

I distinctly remember my neck, shoulders, and back feeling extremely sore, as though I'd stiffened at the impact of a car accident or something. I couldn't explain that. Could it be that during the operation, I'd stiffened up? Maybe I'd lain so completely limp on the operating table that these muscles were stretched? I still don't know. My physical recovery otherwise was much easier than I had expected. The doctors had given me Tylenol with codeine to help with pain, but I didn't need more than one dose; I've been told I have a high threshold for pain. I had little energy for about two days, and I spotted for about twelve days.

My next several weeks went on as normal, except for my weekly visit to the lab for my "hCG quant." I had conceived on March 13, 2011. My molar pregnancy had been diagnosed on May 18, when the pregnancy was eleven weeks, three days gestation. My laboratory results on May 19 showed an hCG level of 43,000. I had my D&C May 20, and a week later, May 27, my hCG level was about 11,000. By June 6 it was already down to 116. My next lab work was taken two weeks later because we had gone out of town, but by June 20, my level was at 19. Another week later, June 29, I was at 13. I skipped a week for travel again, but on July 14 my hCG was at 6, on July 21 it was at 4, and on August 4, which was eleven weeks after my D&C, it was finally less than 2. Now I had only my six-month countdown until I could try to conceive. Each of those months I had my lab tests run, and my hCG thankfully stayed at "zero."

I had a lovely triage nurse from the OB/GYN clinic who would call me with results within twenty-four hours of each test, explaining where we would go from there and asking me if I had any questions or needed anything. She worked closely with the head doctor at the clinic who was in charge of my case. It comforted me to know that another lady in their clinic was going through the same thing. In retrospect perhaps I should have asked the nurse to share my information with this other woman; she and I might have become good friends during this ordeal of ours.

The grief, for me, has come in pieces. I grieve a little each time someone else is pregnant or has a baby because I long to join them. I grieve as I think about how the age gap is growing between my youngest child and her next potential sibling. I grieved when the army moved us away from the people who had loved and supported me in my loss; I wanted them to see me have a healthy baby. I rejoiced at the end of 2011 when I had my last monthly follow-up test at our new army clinic and was cleared to begin trying to conceive again, but I grieved a little each month we weren't able to conceive. It's not that I've been sobbing so much, but I have sadness and a lot of questions. Why did this happen to me? I wonder if doctors will ever find the causes behind molar pregnancies. I'm not sad to the point of depression; I have so much reason for joy in my life, and my faith in God gives me hope. He hasn't answered all my questions, but He has walked with me through my loss.

The grief for my husband has been different. He really surprised me. From the time he discovered I had a molar pregnancy, he was my rock. He listened to me, was my sounding board, and echoed my feelings about how strange it was. My husband is a chaplain in the army, so he is good at being supportive—not because of his job, but because his supportive behavior makes him a great chaplain. No matter how often I wanted to talk about it, he let me. Over a year later, however, while talking with some chaplain peers, a lot of emotions surfaced for him that he hadn't realized were repressed. The stress of leadership during deployment, his return home from service, my nearly immediate pregnancy, and his own feelings after my molar pregnancy had all been set aside; his focus had been caring for me rather than grieving the loss himself, and grieving other losses related to his work. These days he is still my rock, but I also am more inclined to ask how he's doing. Men handle emotions differently, and I accept that. I'm comforted to know that he had emotions stemming from the loss as well—that it was truly a shared experience.

When it comes to talking with our children about things like this, we're very straightforward with them and answer all of their questions the best we can. They knew we were expecting a baby in December and were very excited, thinking ahead to what that might be like and whether it would be a boy or a girl. So we were completely honest about the molar pregnancy the day we found out. They were disappointed, of course, and had as many questions as we did, but they saw that I was still there and well and still their mother. They saw my hope that someday we would try again and shared that hope with me. I have learned through deployments that children take their cues from their parents. If Mom and Dad are confident that the family will get through a deployment and everything will be okay, the children reflect that confidence. On the other hand I am also careful not to appear deceptively stronger than I really am. I share my feelings of sadness and loss with them and listen to their feelings and empathize with them.

Finally, after eight (long) months of trying, in August 2012, we conceived! My anticipation was huge enough to overshadow my concern that this could be another molar pregnancy, although the concern was always there. I made my appointment quickly this time, not wanting to be in suspense about whether this was a viable pregnancy. My new primary care doctor, who was very understanding, expedited the order for an ultrasound, which I had before my first obstetric appointment at the new army hospital. The ultrasound confirmed a healthy baby with a beating heart at six weeks, five days. Surely this time everything would be the healthy pregnancy to which I was accustomed! At my obstetric appointment a week later I met my new doctor, who was also familiar with molar pregnancies and the follow-up needed with a postmolar pregnancy. I was so thankful he understood. He verified a healthy non-molar pregnancy at seven weeks, five days, and sent us home anticipating our next monthly checkup, which would be at twelve weeks.

Unfortunately, at the twelve-week checkup, the doctor could not detect a heartbeat and said that the baby had probably died around ten weeks' gestation. I was heartbroken. This time we had seen a baby. He told me this miscarriage was not my fault in any way and had nothing to do with my previous molar, which I accepted. He did not recommend a D&C, because it is the most invasive approach, so I was medically induced for the miscarriage. The inducement process lasted a couple of weeks, and then I bled and spotted for five more weeks afterward. That experience is another story all on its own.

I understand the risks of a D&C, and I am thankful my doctor preferred to recommend less-invasive means of miscarriage, but this was much harder, because there had been a living child, and because the physical healing process took so much longer. True to his word, my doctor has followed up with pathology testing on the baby I lost as well as hCG testing for my blood to verify that no molar tissue has been triggered to grow. Thankfully, my hCG has dropped quickly, and I don't have to wait six months this time. He only recommends that I wait about two cycles to lessen the risk of an ectopic pregnancy and to allow my body to heal well.

I am now in that healing process. I am thankful for our three healthy girls. I am thankful for supportive family and friends. I am thankful for those who have shared their stories of loss with me, so we can share in our sympathy for one another. I still have a strong desire to add to our family, and I am thankful for a husband who supports that desire. That year, 2011, was the year of the molar, and 2012 was the year of the miscarriage. I hope that 2013 will be the year we have a healthy new baby.

A funny thing happened when I was home for Christmas this past December. I was talking with my paternal grandmother, who expressed her sympathy for my miscarriage. Then she told me that with her first pregnancy, she started bleeding and had gone to the hospital, where the doctor told her there was no baby. She shared with me that she had been relieved that "it had no soul" but had been concerned she would not be able to give her husband the children he wanted. She went on to have four healthy children. I told this story to my own mother later, and she informed me that my maternal grandmother had had a miscarriage with her second pregnancy for which her doctor had said there was no baby.

I was floored! It had been one and half years since my own complete molar pregnancy, and I was just now learning that both of my grandmothers very possibly had had them as well? I am somewhat relieved that it may be genetic and that I am not the only one in my family to experience this, although I doubt my grandmothers were as well informed in the 1940s.

In a way, I am thankful to have experienced these losses. They have allowed me to empathize with many other women who have lost a pregnancy and with people who have experienced other types of losses. Life is messy. Our shared experiences draw us together in community, especially we women. It is comforting to know that we are not the only ones going through this hard time, and it gives us hope to see women often going on to have healthy pregnancies. I hope my story brings you comfort as well.

Chauvonne

My name is Chauvonne, and I am married and the mother of two beautiful girls. I am from Western Australia. On December 4, which is my husband's birthday, we learned that all the trying had paid off—we were going to have another baby to complete our little family! It was the best birthday present I could have given my husband, or so I thought.

Right from the start this pregnancy felt different. I had more pain than usual and I was constantly sick, which I had not been when I was pregnant with the girls, so we thought maybe we were having a boy. For some reason both sides of my abdomen were hurting; the pain got so bad that I was flown to Perth to King Edward Memorial Hospital (KEMH) by the Royal Flying Doctor Service. My husband and daughters drove four hours to be by my side (and because I obviously needed to get home somehow). The doctors at KEMH had no idea why I was having these pains, so after a transvaginal ultrasound and a few more checks I was cleared for the long drive home. The ultrasound showed a very healthy six-weeks-old embryo, and I was so relieved.

Back home, the pain continued for a week or so but then stopped. I had very small spotting at about eight weeks, but I thought nothing of it because it had happened with my other two as well. I also noticed my belly was very large at ten weeks, and I was a little worried that they had missed a baby and maybe there were twins. On February 4, however, I went for my twelve-week scan, and my whole world came crashing down.

We were in the waiting room patiently waiting for our turn, and in walked this frazzled man, late and still trying to get dressed.

"I hope that's not our sonographer," I said to my husband. He laughed and replied that he bet it was. I would have lost that bet! When the man—yes, he was the sonographer—called our name, we followed him to our scan room. He started the ultrasound, and I noticed that when he pushed on my belly it really hurt. He asked if I had had any previous scans, and I told him yes, at KEMH six weeks ago. He then abruptly asked if they had found anything, and my heart sank. I knew then that something was wrong. I looked up at the screen and noticed the baby was tiny for twelve weeks and had no movement at all. The sonographer told us straight out that we had lost the baby and said he was going to call his doctor about what to do next.

When he left I fought back the tears welling in my eyes. My husband went into silent mode and would not even look at me; he shut down right when I needed him most. The sonographer returned and said his doctor could not reach my own doctor because her office wasn't open yet. Our best bet was to wait for the ultrasound results (which would take about two hours!) and then go straight to KEMH and wait in the emergency department. My husband finally said something, but not what I wanted to hear.

"We can't stay in Perth; we have to get home as the dogs will need looking after and we've left the air-conditioning on," he said. I lost the plot with him for thinking the dogs and bloody house were more important to me, but I see now that he was not coping well at all. At the time, I expected him to be my rock, and I was thinking of no one else, including him. I also was so angry with the sonographer for speaking to me rudely that I wanted to sue him. How dare he treat me that way just because he was having a bad day? I didn't say anything to the receptionist, just in case it was my emotions getting to me. It was not until I got into the car that I realized I now had to face my husband's sister and mother who were looking after the girls. This was going to be a hard day. All of my other plans were just put to the back of my mind while all this miscarriage stuff got sorted out.

With our ultrasound results and a doctor's referral in hand we headed back to KEMH. I walked into the emergency department and my heart broke even more because there were pregnant women and babies everywhere. We checked in at reception and waited to be called. While we were waiting my doctor called to see how I was doing and what the ultrasound place had told me to do. She said I was in the right place and that she would call the center to update them on my recent medical history.

When we finally saw the nurse she went over our options to either pass the baby naturally or have a D&C and explained the risks of having another miscarriage. I could tell my husband was thinking we'd have no more babies. I opted for the D&C, because having the baby naturally would mean we'd need to come back to Perth in a week for a follow-up appointment. They scheduled my procedure for the following day, so we headed to my mother-in-law's house, where I cried all afternoon until I fell asleep.

Tuesday morning we returned to KEMH to have this horrible procedure done. I was already sick of everyone saying "Sorry for your loss," and thought if I heard it again I would rip that person's head off. We once again found ourselves in a waiting room full of pregnant women. By the time it was my turn it was about two-thirty in the afternoon and there were still four people waiting after me, two of whom were actually scheduled for the same operating room. I headed in alone, leaving my husband in the waiting room. Not knowing what to expect, I started to get very nervous, but soon I was out cold. Before I knew it I was in recovery and very sore. I was feeling very ill; they even had to give me two doses of antinausea medicine because I was dry heaving and that was making my pain worse. They told me I had lost a bit of blood and would have to stay awhile for monitoring. I dozed in and out, unaware of how much time was passing. Finally I was wheeled out on my stretcher to wait for my husband. He came in with the most worried look on his face, but it vanished when he saw me. He said I had been gone so long that he had watched a whole movie, and when it finished and I wasn't out yet he had begun to wonder what was going on. I asked him the time, and he said it was nearly six o'clock. The doctor who had done the procedure arrived and told us that my placenta had been very bulky and had taken longer to remove than expected. The doctor also said that I had lost a lot of blood and that I wasn't to do anything for the next few weeks. We finally left the hospital at seven-thirty and went straight home to bed.

At home the next day, my husband put me on couch arrest and did everything for me and the girls. I did not know what to feel. I felt hurt, angry, and confused, but most of all I felt empty, as though something were missing. People wanted to visit, but I shut down. I didn't answer the phone, e-mails, or text messages. I just wanted to crawl under a rock and stay there until everyone forgot about it. I was sick of seeing everyone's looks of pity; they just made things worse. I wasn't feeling any better physically either; in fact, three days later (Friday, February 8), I was in excruciating pain. I thought I'd search Google to see if it was normal or if something was wrong, but I could not get a clear answer so I phoned health direct. They told me to go to my local hospital straight away.

When we got there my own doctor was away, so we had a different doctor who knew nothing of my history. He said it looked as though they had perforated a fallopian tube, and there was probably blood in it. He gave me tramadol because I can't take codeine and sent me home. The next Monday my grandmother, whom I had missed catching up with the week before because of the ultrasound, passed away, and I now had to deal with losing both my baby and my most favorite person in the whole world. I didn't think it could possibly get any worse.

The pain had persisted for ten days, and I had been thru two packets of tramadol with no effect. I returned to my local hospital on Friday, February 15, and was assigned a wonderful nurse who gave me an injection for the pain and told me to head straight for KEMH or Joondalup Hospital. I went home and told my husband that we had to go back to Perth because something was wrong, and once again he shut down. We didn't leave for Perth until the next afternoon, and once there I waited until the following day to go to the hospital when there would be more staff available. I decided to go to Joondalup instead of KEMH because it was closer to where we were staying and easier for my husband and sister-in-law to swap spots without leaving her partner alone with five kids under age five for too long. My sister-in-law came with me first, driving me to the hospital while our partners looked after our children. We were in the waiting room for quite some time.

When they took be back to be examined they felt around my abdomen and decided to do an internal exam. They gave me morphine before the internal because I was in so much pain. When the results came back from the lab they showed I had an infection. The doctors wanted to keep me in overnight, but I refused because the next day was my grandmother's funeral, and I wasn't missing my chance to say goodbye. So instead they ran an intravenous line of antibiotics through my system and gave me prescriptions for more antibiotics and painkillers to take home. I had had enough of this whole year and just wanted it to be over already.

February 17 was a horrible day. I felt so lost at the funeral; my cousin, who was due to give birth the same day I had been, was there and it was very difficult to keep it together. I somehow got through the church service without losing control. On our drive to the cemetery I was thinking, "This is it. There is nothing else God can throw at me that I can't handle." At that moment, my phone rang. The caller was the doctor who had performed my D&C. He was calling to tell me that it had been a partial molar pregnancy and that I'd have to go to them or my local doctor for blood tests. He said my doctor would be able to advise me from there.

After a very long weekend, we were finally home. I wanted to learn everything I could about molar pregnancies, but I was too scared to look them up. I asked my friend to check Google before me to see if I'd be able to handle the results. She came back with somewhat good news but told me to be cautious when reading. She said there were two types of molar pregnancy, and although mine was the least horrible of the two it still wasn't nice. Over the next few weeks I searched Google for all the information I could find about partial molar pregnancies. A few times I came across things I didn't want to hear, so I'd scare myself out of searching for a while, but after a few days I'd find another question I needed to answer. I had too much time on my hands to dwell on things. I had no baby and wanted—needed—one badly, but I had to wait with no idea how long.

Things at home had gotten so bad that the kids were getting yelled at for no reason and my husband and I were constantly fighting. You could cut the tension with a knife. I even searched Google at one point to find out how many pills I needed to take to end my life, which was not like me at all. Around this time I started to read forum messages from other women going through the same things, and I also joined a few Facebook support groups. I came to realize there was hope. I had had three tests so far, and my level was down to 27. My husband finally opened up to me and explained that he didn't want to try again because he didn't want to see me go through all of it again. My moods slowly improved; I wasn't so snappy and on edge all the time. For the first time in weeks I was enjoying people's company again and laughing with my kids.

My numbers kept going down over the following weeks, going from 27 to 6, 4, 2, and then 1. At eight weeks I had stayed at 1, but my doctor wasn't sure what was considered negative was so I called KEMH. They confirmed that I was finally negative. Woo Hoo! I was finally negative and back to my normal self. My husband was still in doubt about trying again so I did more Google searching and finally found the results I wanted to hear. Dr. Goldstein, a molar pregnancy expert in the United States, had said that as long as you have been negative for three consecutive weeks, your molar pregnancy was over. THANK HEAVEN! I gave my husband the good news and some more information to read. I'm supposed to wait three to six months before getting pregnant again, and I am scared, nervous, and excited all at the same time, but I figure I'm so much stronger than I was before, so I CAN DO THIS!

Courtney

My husband and I met during our undergraduate years and were married when I was twenty-four and he was twenty-seven. At that time, we agreed that children were in our future plans, but we were in no rush. Shortly after our marriage, we bought our first home and invested a lot of time and energy in our fixer-upper. I started graduate school at the age of twenty-seven, and during that four-year time span there were many ups and downs that came with the stress of being a full-time doctoral student, the responsibilities of being a homeowner, and my new role as a wife. We got through it, however, and my husband was always there for me and supportive through it all. He was like some kind of saint, my rock through very challenging and exhausting times.

By my third year in the program, and just before my thirtieth birthday, my biological clock started ticking. More and more often my thoughts were turning toward starting a family. Truth is, my husband had wanted to start a family years before I did, but my graduate studies had taken priority, and I felt a great deal of guilt about this. I didn't want to keep him waiting any longer, so we decided that after I graduated in August 2011 we would begin trying. After spending more than a decade using birth control pills, I stopped taking them in the spring of 2011. That summer, I finished my dissertation and trudged through my final months as a doctoral candidate. It was a very exciting, busy, and somewhat hectic time. To celebrate my graduation, my husband set aside his prior year's Christmas bonus, and we took our first true vacation—a trip to Hawaii. It was then that we officially started trying to conceive. Aside from taking prenatal vitamins for a couple of months, I paid no attention to my preconception health. Within a few months we were pregnant. It was almost too easy.

Just before Thanksgiving, on November 20, 2011, my period was two days late. I went to the drug store and picked up a test. It was positive! We were happy and a little nervous. We figured out the estimated due date, which was July 25, and began dreaming about this baby. Although part of me was cautious and wanted to keep our news secret, I did share with my mother and sister that we were expecting. With the impending holiday, I knew I wouldn't be able to keep my excitement concealed, so I asked my husband to break the news. During the blessing of the meal at Thanksgiving dinner, we all shared something we were thankful for, and when it came to my husband, he exclaimed that he was "thankful that we were going to be parents." Everyone was so excited, and in that moment I was blissfully unaware of what was to come. I often think back to that brief moment, when I was still full of joy and wonder, still optimistic and carefree. Other than extreme exhaustion, I felt fine; I had had no morning sickness or crazy pregnancy symptoms, I was just very tired and usually in bed by eight o'clock. The Monday after Thanksgiving, I felt like I was coming down with something. I sneezed a lot that day and had a fever with chills that evening. My husband had pulled out the Christmas tree and the decorations, but all I could do after work was nap on the couch and watch him start decorating. As I lay there the song, "All I Want for Christmas" came on the radio. Even though Mariah Carey annoys me, I sang along and rubbed my belly, because all I wanted for Christmas was for this baby to grow and be healthy. I loved it so much already.

A few days later—about six weeks into the pregnancy—I knew something wasn't right. It began one night with a sharp, tugging pain on the left side of my uterus that lasted about thirty seconds. It took my breath away, so much so that I gasped and my husband called to me from the next room, "Are you okay?" I assured him I was fine; it was just a cramp that caught me off guard. It was a very strange feeling, but I tried my best to shake it off and not overanalyze. The next day, I was consulting in a classroom and had to excuse myself for yet another bathroom break. At that point in the pregnancy, urination was much more frequent. This time, however, when I wiped, I saw awful brown spotting on the tissue. *This isn't good*, I thought. Immediately, fear hit me and my head spun. I fixed my gaze on one of the bright blue tiles in the bathroom, told myself to get it together, and took a few deep breaths. The sound of elementary students leaving the cafeteria was just outside the bathroom door, and I waited for them to pass before leaving. I didn't want them to see the terror on my face. I gathered myself before going back to the classroom.

That brown spotting continued through the next week. At first I did my best to redirect the negative thoughts, rationally reminding myself that based on my research, spotting can be common in early pregnancy, and "brown blood is old blood" that apparently is better than red blood. Yet logic didn't change the deep-down fear that I was losing this pregnancy. The spotting would let up and hope would return, but then a few hours later the spotting would resume. I called the doctor, but she couldn't see me any earlier and said to keep the appointment I had already scheduled in a few days.

Two days before my first appointment, I was in the bathroom and found the spotting had returned. I had this heavy, sinking feeling of knowing that I wasn't having a baby. I cried—oh, how I sobbed! I couldn't hold back the fear anymore. When my husband came home from work that night, I shared my fears that I had lost the baby. He comforted me and reminded me that there was nothing we could do at that point and that worrying would not change anything. *What will be, will be* were his words.

At the ultrasound a few days later (December 7), I told my doctor about the spotting. My husband sat patiently through my annual exam portion, and once that was done the ultrasound began. As she began the ultrasound, she explained that she would be looking for "a white spot" on the screen. What felt like an eternity passed as she scanned, and still she hadn't found anything. I craned my neck to see the screen, so much so that I pulled a muscle in my neck, but still nothing. She kept looking, explaining that it could take a few minutes to find. She double-checked my cycle dates, which I assured her were accurate. There was no way I was earlier than seven weeks, and I believed that I was in fact closer to eight weeks. All she could find, however, was "a black sac."

At that moment, all of my fears were justified. I struggled to hold back the trembling lip and tears, but soon I started crying. She mentioned something about "a fetal sac, but no pole…probably chromosomal abnormalities…I don't want to give you false hope, it doesn't look like a good pregnancy." I don't remember everything she said in those minutes, but I do remember that she hugged me and said she was sorry. My poor husband just sat there, watching the horror unfold. She told us to take as long as we needed in the room and then to come have my blood drawn when I was ready. I gathered myself, got dressed, and my husband consoled me.

Sitting down to have my blood drawn, I warned the nurse that I hated needles. She pointed to the wall next to the station that was filled with hundreds of pictures of babies delivered by my doctor, and their smiling families. "Well, here are lots of pictures you can look at instead," she said. I directed my gaze to the tray of needles, bandages, and vials. At that point, I was holding back the tears, and the last thing I could look at was all those darling babies! That wall of babies was one of the hardest things about the weekly blood draws that were yet to come. I hated seeing all those happy families and their precious babies while I was being pricked and prodded.

My husband drove home from the appointment, and I cried. What did I do wrong? What happened? Unfortunately there were no answers. My parents knew about my ultrasound and wanted to know how it went, but I hardly understood it myself, let alone well enough to explain to my family. The day after the ultrasound, I was numb. I cancelled my work appointment and didn't really leave the bed except perhaps twice. I cried a little, but mostly I felt empty, like a void, a vacuum of emotion. My doctor called to report that my hCG level came back at 28,258, which she said was high for a missed miscarriage at eight weeks. She asked me to come back the next day (December 9) for a blood draw, which showed my hCG at 39,824. She scheduled me for further blood work on December 13 and reminded me of the prescription for Tylenol 3 for "when the pain and cramps start." I explained, "Nothing is happening... there is no pain and I'm not passing anything." In the meantime, I had work obligations to fulfill, appointments and staff trainings that couldn't be rescheduled. At each training and each consultation visit I wondered: *will this be the day that the miscarriage starts?* Not only was I losing the pregnancy, I had no control over when it would start, and I had this horrible vision of the bleeding starting in the middle of a staff training. Because of this, I shared with my fellow training colleagues what was happening, just in case. Of course, that raised more questions for which I had no answers.

When I returned to the doctor for a third blood draw, I described that I had had some cramping and had passed a small, quarter-sized clot over the weekend, but I still hadn't really passed much tissue. She did an exam and said my cervix was dilated to one centimeter, which was probably causing the pain. They drew my blood and called me the next day, saying that the most recent hCG level was now at 88,000. My doctor asked me to come for another ultrasound on December 16, 2011. In the meantime, I scoured my pregnancy books and the Internet trying to figure out what in the hell was happening to me. The first time I saw the term *molar pregnancy* was in a book my husband got me for my birthday that year, *What to Expect When You Are Expecting*. The condition received a scant paragraph, and to be honest, this was the last thing I was "expecting." So I logged on to the university's online library and began searching for scholarly papers to find out more about this "molar pregnancy."

When I went in for my second ultrasound, the image on the screen had changed to a dark mass of clusters. It almost looked like Swiss cheese.

"I think it is a molar pregnancy," my doctor said.

"Why?" I asked. "Due to the rising hCG and that strange image on the ultrasound?"

She looked surprised, so I explained that I had been using my research skills over the past few weeks and that finding scientific papers had been the only way I had any semblance of control in the situation.

That day, she took a final blood draw to measure my hCG, which had increased to 117,000, and she scheduled my D&C for December 20. For the first time in my life, I missed my family's annual cookie baking because I was preparing for surgery and was in too much physical and emotional pain. In those last few days before the D&C, my abdomen became extremely distended, much larger than that of a woman carrying a healthy nine-week pregnancy. It felt sore and heavy, and walking was uncomfortable, so I stayed reclined. I was angry with the invader in my body and afraid it would turn into cancer. I couldn't do much but lay on the couch on those days between the D&C and Christmas. I did my best to put on a smile and go to all the holiday celebrations, but really I just wanted to be at home in bed. Christmas was ruined.

In the midst of the medical process that was unfolding, I received an offer to teach at the university. I was hesitant to commit to the assignment, unsure of what the next few months would hold. *Would I need chemo? If so, would I become too sick to teach?* Yet I also saw it as a great opportunity to continue developing my career as a recently graduated Ph.D., and in the back of my mind I knew it also would be an excellent distraction, which was what I desperately wanted. I needed something to take my mind off of what was happening. I agreed to the assignment and began preparing for my first quarter as an adjunct professor. I focused one hundred percent on work, and anytime the thought of cancer crept into my mind, I focused on my teaching or read a paper about molar pregnancies, papers with objective data that I could use to reel me back in with logic.

To complement my reading, I also joined an online group for molar pregnancy support on babycenter.com. Establishing that connection gave me an outlet where I could find other women at different stages in their journey, from those like me who were recently diagnosed to those who were healed and trying again and even those who had gone on to have healthy pregnancies. Women whom I had never met were there to encourage me and to commiserate with me when I was struggling through very difficult times. I don't know where I would be today without that group and the friends I have made. I was no longer suffering this obscure condition alone. No one in my "real life" had ever heard of a molar pregnancy. No one understood that it was so much more than a pregnancy loss; it was the loss of a dream, a loss of pregnancy innocence, a feeling of being tricked by my body, and a fear of complications, chemotherapy, and ongoing blood draws.

During my follow-up, my doctor recommended birth control. I told her I was not comfortable going back on the pill and that I had had a tough hormonal transition when I had gone off of it after twelve years. I was not willing to go back on, particularly not while pregnancy hormones were still running rampant in my body. I assured her that we would use condoms during my follow-up period. My weekly blood draws started one week after my D&C, on December 27, and the first draw looked promising: hCG 2,840. They continued to drop; two weeks later (January 4) my hCG was at 450. By three weeks (January 11) it was down to ninety-seven, and at four weeks (January 18) it was thirty-two. This brought a huge sigh of relief, because research shows that this rate of decline correlates with a significant decrease in odds of recurrence. By five weeks (January 24) my hCG was 12; at six weeks (February 1) it was 6; and by seven weeks (February 8) it was 3. I was finally negative! At the eight-week draw (February 14), it stayed low at 2, and at nine weeks (February 22) it was down to 1. Monthly draws were all that were required after that. On March 21 my hCG was still 1, and on April 18 and again on May 21 it was less than 1.

In the scheme of things, I had an ideal recovery, physically. My doctor kept on top of my diagnosis and management, which is a different experience than some other women have had based on what I have heard from my support group board. My doctor also did a phenomenal job with the D&C; I felt better the moment I woke from anesthesia and had no difficulty in recovery. She did a thorough job with the evacuation, as evidenced by my not requiring a second D&C, as some molar pregnancy patients have had to endure. I believe the early ultrasound and her responsive tracking of my blood work allowed for early detection and effective evacuation, which helped to prevent recurrence of invasive GTD.

Despite the swift physical recovery, the months during the blood work follow-up were pretty rough, emotionally speaking. I am generally an optimistic, hard-working person who is social and outgoing. Yet during that time, I started to feel like a completely different person. Most days, I felt like a zombie just going through the motions. I lost focus and energy and was more overwhelmed with daily life. Once the fear of chemo had passed, I was left to deal with the pain of the loss. I had this misconception that once I cleared the hurdle of recurrence, things would just return to normal and I would bounce back to the person that I once was. It was difficult coming to the realization that I wasn't going to get back to my old "normal," that this experience had changed me. It would be months before I could see how it had strengthened me, and I was stuck in that place where the fear of chemotherapy was gone but I was still grappling with the sadness of loss. Beyond the sadness aspect, I physically became much more fatigued and displayed symptoms of hypothyroid. Blood tests would later reveal that my thyroid and adrenals were not functioning optimally, which I believe was triggered by the molar pregnancy.

In June 2012, we started trying again for a pregnancy. This time, I was prepared. I had been tracking my cycles using fertilityfriend.com (e.g., tracking basal body temperature and observing cervical mucus) since January 2012. This data showed me that my cycles were ovulatory and gave me a good idea of when to expect ovulation. Another area in which I better prepared was dental health. At the start of June, I had some old amalgam fillings removed and replaced with composite at the dentist's recommendation, because they were breaking down. I took care of that business and was excited for the return of my husband—who was out of town on a business trip for two weeks—so that we could start trying again. On July 1 I had a positive pregnancy test. That day I gave my husband a belated birthday present, a light-hearted book about being a dad, along with the positive test. We had a moment of brief excitement, but based on our history I wasn't banking too much on the positive test. I took a test every day, and I watched that pink line fade. My period came two days late that cycle, and as the line faded, we sadly realized that we were experiencing an early loss, or a "chemical pregnancy" as it is commonly called. I was monitored at my doctor's office, and my hCG was less than 1 about a week later. Boy was I angry that week! Regardless, however, I wanted to keep trying, so that is what we did.

The following month I continued to track my cycles and started reading up more on prenatal nutrition. *Real Food for Mother and Baby* introduced me to traditional diets and the work of Weston A. Price. I started reading everything I could on the topic and began to adopt changes to my diet accordingly. Meanwhile, my husband and I continued to try for pregnancy, and at the end of the month we went on a vacation that I had conveniently scheduled for the estimated due date of our molar pregnancy. On that vacation, I spent time with my sister and her partner, my mom, aunts, and uncle on the West coast. It was a great trip. We spent time at a beach house on the shore, I got quality time with my family, and I didn't think once about that due date. Upon returning from vacation, I took a pregnancy test the very first morning. It was positive again, but then I watched it fade again over the next few days—another chemical pregnancy. My hCG monitoring showed that my level returned to negative within ten days.

Ever since we started trying to have a baby, I have been acutely aware of the many friends and family around us that are conceiving. It has been a sensitive topic for me, but one that I can finally say no longer causes pain. The week that I learned of our loss, back in December 2011, a friend from college and then a former coworker both gave birth to sweet baby boys. I saw their updates on Facebook, and although I was happy for them, I would be lying if I didn't admit that it hurt to see those newborns. It was hard to separate the pain of my loss, just having learned of the molar pregnancy. I wanted a little boy of my own so badly! As summer rolled around, many more friends were announcing pregnancies, but those announcements and newborns just depressed me. It seemed as though so many ladies around me were pregnant, many with their second or even third child, yet here I was, still wondering when our time would come. In August I was at a friend's bachelorette party, and one of our friends brought her newborn baby to the shower. Her baby was born right around my original due date. Some of the girls were taking turns holding the baby, and every time I looked at that newborn, all I could think was how I should have one of my own, just that size. Almost ironically, someone asked me "So, are you planning to have kids?" I choked. All I could say was, "Yes, we are, but it hasn't happened yet."

The frustration and defeat I felt at that point was heavy. Somehow, though, we kept trying. Over the next couple of months there were no positive tests. Although we weren't dealing with the repeated losses, I started to wonder what was wrong with me. Why these trends of failure? All my life, I have been able to set a goal, work toward it, problem solve as needed, and eventually meet the goal. This woman who put herself through college on scholarship, who married the man of her dreams, who bought a home, studied at university, and even achieved a doctorate was now failing at one thing that comes naturally—and often unplanned—to countless women. It sent me into a deep depression. After much soul searching and talking with my husband, we agreed that the stress of conceiving was too much for both of us. We decided to take a break, to take a different approach to trying. I let go of my perfectly planned two babies and the dream of having our children before I turned thirty-five. I decided instead to focus on my health, which was perhaps the lesson in all of this. Maybe

I needed to focus on getting to my optimal health before trying to bring our first child into this world.

Data from my ongoing charts showed some potential problems, with excessive spotting and lower basal body temperatures. After blood work at my primary care physician showed some endocrine abnormalities, I was referred to an endocrinologist. Her testing confirmed I had low thyroid and adrenal function as well as a nontoxic thyroid nodule. I have researched the treatment options and, at this time, I am using an alternative nonpharmaceutical intervention that focuses largely on diet and supplements. We have maintained our break from trying to conceive, and as of January 2013 I have finally had all of the amalgams replaced and have completed all of the recommended dental work. I am continuing with diet and lifestyle changes that promote fertility. My husband is as well. We both needed a break from the stress of repeated losses and failure to conceive.

My husband has recently started a new job, and we are planning to start trying again in the fall of 2013. My hope is that focused efforts and time to heal—both physically and emotionally—will make a difference in our next try. Despite our difficult journey, I have faith that we will eventually grow our family. It may not be on the timeline I originally conceived, and it may not be the idyllic "one boy and one girl" that we dreamed of, but we are okay with that. If it takes us years to get one, boy or girl, we will love that baby more than it will ever understand. If we somehow get lucky enough to have two, well, that will just be wonderful.

Halina

In June 2010 my partner of eight years and I decided to try again for a baby. We had been trying on and off since 2007 after having a miscarriage, but this time we decided I would fully come off of the pill. Months and months went by. My periods were not coming on, so each month I would have the same hopeful thought: "I'm pregnant...I must be!" Yet each test I took came back negative. I knew it might take a while for the birth control to clear out of my system, so I carried on with trying and testing and just hoped that one day I would see the positive sign instead of the negative.

After eleven months of trying and still having neither periods nor a positive test, I made an appointment with my doctor and was diagnosed with polycystic ovary syndrome. She explained that this may make it difficult to become pregnant but that I should keep trying. (It used to make me so angry when she would say that, as though I were baking a cake or something. Keep trying and eventually it will be perfect!)

I went back to the doctor again after a few months had gone by. I had been trying for fifteen months without success. This time they took me seriously and said I probably would need some help getting pregnant. Finally I was getting somewhere! I was waiting for the letter scheduling my appointment at the fertility clinic when one day my auntie asked how I was getting on with it all. I explained the story to her, and then out the blue she said, "I think you are pregnant. I just have a feeling." I told her I couldn't be and that the doctor had told me it was unlikely to happen naturally. She insisted I take a test anyway.

The next day I got a test. I wasn't nervous in the slightest, because this was probably the hundredth test I'd taken in the past fifteen months. This time, however—much to my surprise—it was positive! My eyes filled with tears. I could not believe that after so many long months it finally had happened. I was pregnant—I was going to be a mum! My partner was as excited as I was. That night we just kept rubbing my tummy, which did seem a little large, but we thought perhaps I was farther along than I had guessed.

The next morning the sickness started. It was awful. From seven until eight-thirty I was constantly sick; then again at lunch time; and then again in the evening from six until roughly ten o'clock every day and every night. This being my first proper pregnancy, I just thought it was normal.

I had a scan scheduled for September 16, 2011. We both were so excited; the days leading up to it felt as though they dragged forever! The day finally came, but as we sat in the waiting room a sudden fear came over me. What if I lose the baby again? What if they don't find a heartbeat? My partner tried to reassure me that everything would be okay, but I was petrified.

"Halina, would you like to come through?" a lovely midwife named Holly asked. She brought us to the exam room and explained that the ultrasound technician would be with me in a minute. I lay on the bed and the technician came in, but she didn't look too friendly and didn't say much. I explained that I didn't know how far along I was because I didn't have period dates to go by. She just nodded and carried on rubbing my belly and looking at the screen. I knew something was wrong. Tears started rolling down my cheeks. She explained that all she could see was the sac but no baby, but she said that that could be because I was too early. I already had a belly bump, however, so in my mind it didn't add up.

Holly, the midwife, explained that sometimes this could happen and that the next scan could be perfectly fine. I was booked in again for October 6. Every day leading up to it I was getting more and more sick; the smell of food made me vomit and the exhaustion was ridiculous. I felt as though I were dying.

October 6 arrived and once again Holly called me in. A different technician did the ultrasound this time, and when I lifted my top up she said "Ooh, a nice little bump we should be able to see a baby today!" She started the scan and straight away I could hear a beating rhythm. "There you go," she said. "That's your little baby's heartbeat!" Those words and that sound will forever stay in my heart. I asked if everything looked okay. "Yes," she responded. "That's a very healthy quick heartbeat there. I can say you are six weeks, five days, and due 28 May 2012." Looking at the screen I couldn't make out the baby shape but I didn't care—it was my baby with a heartbeat and that's all that mattered! "Can I have a photo please?" I asked. She laughed. "Not much to see, but of course you can."

My next scan would be on November 16, at twelve weeks. That's when my life changed forever.

Through the weeks leading up to my next scan I was okay except for the continued sickness and exhaustion. I was loving my pregnancy, watching my belly get bigger each week and taking photos of my ever-growing bump! Then the cravings started. I loved that part—it made me properly feel pregnant. I found myself wanting things I didn't normally like. One craving I had was for milk—I drank glasses and glasses of it every day. I loved all of these "pregnancy things." At about nine weeks I had this strange feeling in my tummy almost as though I were going down a hill quickly in the car. When I spoke to my mum about it, she explained could be the baby moving. I only had that feeling once, but it was the best thing ever.

November 16 came, and I was so excited about seeing a proper baby figure on the monitor. We waited patiently for my name to be called. Holly was there again to take us back, and I felt reassured that it was someone I had previously seen. I went with my partner and mum into the room and lay down with my shirt rolled up and waited to see the image. This time when the technician pressed the scanner on me I knew straight away something wasn't quite right. It seemed to take ages to pick anything up. I was looking at the screen praying and hoping that I would see something, anything, and then I did—except it wasn't what I had hoped for. "I'm sorry," the technician said. "The baby doesn't have a heartbeat; you have had a missed miscarriage. The baby is the size of an eight-week pregnancy, not twelve-week."

To be honest, the next few hours are a complete blur. I don't remember much except for the doctor saying that I needed a D&C but that it could be a few days' wait. I had already had one dead baby in me for four weeks; I just wanted this one out of me. The thought of keeping it made me physically sick. Fortunately, they managed to get me a bed the very next day. We requested an autopsy of the fetus to see what had happened and to try to get some answers. We were told that the results could take up to two weeks to come through.

I remember going home and thinking "I can't wait until tomorrow; I need it out of me now." Something I had loved so much with all of my heart was gone. I remember sitting on the sofa with my partner and crying for about two hours solid. I could not believe my miracle baby was gone. All that time I had thought I would be fine, but my body had known otherwise. Why me? What have I done to deserve this?

We then had the dreaded task of telling friends and family the news. Everyone said how sorry they were, but they just did not seem to understand. All they kept saying was, "Maybe it's for the best" or "You're still young, you have plenty of time to try again." I was sick to death of hearing those things! So what if I was young? That didn't give anyone the right to take it away from me. I was getting to the point where if I heard those words again I was going to blow! Others said things like "Well, give it a few months you can try again." I did not want another baby, I wanted *that* one! People who have never experienced a miscarriage don't seem to know what to say. In truth, I sometimes wished they hadn't said anything at all.

The next morning went to the local hospital for the D&C. I remember waking up and feeling empty. My tummy felt as though everything had been ripped out, and the pain was unreal. I was so sore I couldn't even walk. The nurse came to help me get dressed, and I saw blood everywhere. I just cried and cried. The nurse said the blood was completely normal and that it would stop within a few days. She was so lovely and understanding; I wish they were all like that! Finally the consultant came to discharge me and said that I had bled quite a bit more than expected and that if it carried I should come straight back to the hospital.

Days went by and I still was in agony. I couldn't sit down because everything was sore and I was still bleeding. A week had passed still it didn't ease, so I went back to the hospital and explained everything to the nurse. Then the consultant who had done the D&C came in. "Your blood results and autopsy results have come back," he said. "You have had a rare type of pregnancy that we call a hydatidiform mole. You could need medication to treat this."

I didn't quite understand what he was going on about. He explained that my hCG level was very high, 40,000, when really it should be at zero. He was being very careful about explaining everything; I think he was afraid of scaring me. I brought up the bit about medication again. "We use something which is the same to treat cancer," he explained. "But I'm not saying you have cancer, because you don't. So please don't think you have cancer." He said that I would get a letter in the mail with more information and that I would be referred to Charing Cross Hospital in London for further blood tests.

After that I had to see another consultant who had dealt with molar pregnancy patients before and who would try to explain what would happen next. His English was not very good, however, which was troubling enough, but then he said the scariest thing I'd ever heard. He said that yes, I did have a tumor, and yes, I would need chemotherapy if the tumor did not go away by itself. I also had to have my lungs x-rayed to see if the cancer had spread to them.

Cancer?! Hang on a minute—no one had said anything about tumors or cancer! He was blunt with his answers and told me that in most cases this tumor did turn to cancer. I was so confused; he was telling me I had cancer, and in my mind I thought was dying. (It wasn't until after doing my own research that I learned molar pregnancies are not cancer straight away. This doctor had gotten it completely wrong and scared the hell out of me!)

All of this seemed too much for me to handle. I cried uncontrollably and started having severe panic attacks and trouble sleeping. I just wanted to crawl up in a ball. I was grieving my baby plus dealing with the thought of this "tumor" in me. People didn't understand what it was or how I felt, not even friends and family. Only my partner understood, but even he seemed to be getting on with life, so I soon decided to go to counseling. Charing Cross has a counselor who works specifically with women who have had molar pregnancies. I saw her every week for six weeks, and I can honestly say she saved my life.

In the meantime my first sample box came through the mail, and every Friday morning I had to go down to my local hospital to do the blood test. I had the same lady each time, which made it easier; I didn't have to explain every time why I was there. Then on the Tuesday after, I would ring Charing Cross for my results. The first week my hCG went down really quickly, dropping from 40,000 to eighty-eight. It then dropped to 64, 50, 44, 21, and 6 over subsequent tests. It stayed at 6 for three weeks, and then finally fell to zero. The lady on the phone told me that if it had taken two more weeks to get to zero I would most likely have needed chemotherapy.

Getting that zero was such an amazing feeling. I knew I still needed to do urine samples for another six months, but those were just once a month rather than every week. Trying to explain that feeling to someone who did not understand was so difficult. In my mind I was all-clear; I didn't have a tumor in me anymore. Things were slowly getting back to normal.

It was March 2012, and I knew May 28 (my due date) was quickly approaching. I was dreading it. My counselor suggested naming our baby as a way to help with the grieving process, so we named her Holly May. We decided on Holly after the midwife who had looked after me and because it all happened close to Christmas, and on May because that had been my due month. It seemed the perfect name—Holly May, our little girl. (We didn't actually know the sex, but I always had a feeling it would be a girl.)

In August 2012 I got my all-clear letter, and we were ready to try again. As of now, January 2013, I still have not fallen pregnant. I am having problems again with my periods, so we are waiting for a hospital appointment to see if we can undergo fertility treatment. These past few years have been the scariest time of my life and also the saddest, but yet all this also has made me stronger. I cannot express how much my partner has been there for me, listening and holding my hand every step of the way. I still get sad days in which I am filled with emotion, especially if I hear someone is expecting. If I go into shops and see cute baby outfits I still get that lump in my throat, and I think I always will. When that happens, though, I think to myself that Holly May is looking down on me, and that seems to get me through.

Now that I have gotten through all of the "hard" dates—my due date anniversary and my first Christmas—I feel like the worst is over. With the help of my partner, I managed to get through them. I will forever miss my miracle baby; no matter how many children I have, she will always be my special angel watching over me.

On one of my down days I found this quote and even now I think of it and it seems to help:

> "After every chapter in life there is a new chapter waiting to begin, after every sadness there is always a bit of happiness, and after every storm there is always a ray of sunshine."

Jennifer

During the summer of 2011, I was employed in my first teaching job out of college. This was my first job where I had benefits, so my husband and I started trying to have a baby immediately (we had wanted one for a while, but did not have the insurance or money to cover the pregnancy expenses). After stopping my birth control in June, I did not have regular periods, but the doctor told me that that was normal. In January, it had been four months since my last period (no period usually means no ovulation), so the doctor gave me medroxy-progesterone to induce a period, hoping to "jump start" my system. I had a period after taking the medicine, but no more after that. In March, the doctor decided to try again, so I took another round of medication and had another period.

After a trip to the Smoky Mountains the first week of June, I still had not had a period, and my breasts were killing me. I thought I was just tired from the trip, but when the feeling didn't go away, I took a pregnancy test. It was positive! I thought all my prayers had been answered. We had just bought a new house, so I began picking out colors for the baby's room and told the family. Everyone was so excited. This would be my parents' first grandchild! I called my doctor, but he was on sabbatical during the summer, so I called a different doctor who had been highly recommended by people in the area. The office staff set up an appointment for my first ultrasound at the end of July. We bought a baby journal, ordered a crib for the new house, and painted the nursery. I will never forget how incredibly happy I was. For once in my life, everything seemed to be coming together.

In July 2012 I had an eight-day training for my new teaching position. I was so excited to be teaching in the town I lived in, and I would no longer have a long commute every day. During the training, I found it very hard to sit up on the laboratory stools and participate as I normally would. I was just so incredibly tired and hungry. I had been taking naps every day, and a full day's activity now drained me more than I realized. During the second week of training I went to the washroom and passed a little clot. It scared me to death. On the commute home I called my sister-in-law, who is a nurse. She got me calmed down (and probably saved my life, because I was driving on a busy interstate) but recommended that I go to the emergency room for an ultrasound. So after I got home, my husband and I drove to the emergency room, where we waited anxiously for two hours.

As he did the ultrasound, the technician could not see anything, so he switched to a transvaginal ultrasound. I heard nothing, and he had the monitor turned away from me. I asked him what was happening, but he said he was not allowed to tell me anything. Finally, after I was taken back to my room, the doctor showed up. He told me I had had a miscarriage and that I needed to follow up with my obstetrician the next day. I cannot describe the pain that went through me at that moment. I was numb; I couldn't process what he was telling me. Sitting here writing this, seven months later, I am still breaking into tears.

The next morning I called the doctor's office, and they squeezed me in that afternoon. They did their own ultrasound and sent me for blood work. I was there all day, most of the time sitting in the waiting room with happy mothers and their babies or their huge pregnant stomachs. Jealousy ran through me, and everything just felt so unfair. I began to think about the clot that I passed. Was that my baby? Did I flush my baby? Finally I was called back to see the doctor. Dr. P asked what the emergency room doctor had told me, and I said that he had confirmed a miscarriage. She then showed me the ultrasound films. There were all of these grape-like clusters everywhere. Dr. P told me that I had had a complete molar pregnancy. She was so kind and explained everything, cried with me, and discussed options. She told me the clusters I saw on the ultrasound were tumors created by the mole. They had posed as a pregnancy and fed off the pregnancy hormone in my uterus. There was an urgent need for a D&C to remove these tumors before they turned cancerous. After talking, we estimated that I was six to eight weeks pregnant, but my hCG level was way over 100,000, which was extremely high. She asked if I was up for surgery the next morning. I told her yes, and away I went for presurgery laboratory work and registration. My family came in from Kentucky to support me, which meant a lot, but at the time I was so numb I couldn't process anything or stop crying. The next day after surgery the doctor said everything had gone well, so they scheduled me for weekly appointments to monitor my condition and hCG levels.

We moved into the new house the next week. I couldn't help, because of the surgery. I tried to go on with normal life, but how could I? This big, empty house with the "baby" room, which my husband had quickly changed to a gym, was a constant reminder of everything I had lost—or didn't even really have to begin with. This is the cruelest disease I have ever heard of, maybe if I had known this was a possibility it would not have felt so unreal at the time. I still look at that room and feel sad.

It took ten weekly visits to the doctor before my hCG level came down. I had muscle pain and cramping from the surgery for three to four weeks. I still have trouble sleeping at night. My level has stayed down at zero, and I only have to be monitored monthly now. Being on birth control again is no fun. There is not a day that goes by that I do not think about a baby.

The chances of the molar repeating if I get pregnant within a year are too high to risk. After reading information online and listening to my doctor, we still have no idea why this happened to us. That is the saddest thing about this disease: it is so rare that no one bothers researching it. If I could have done anything to prevent it I would have. I wish there were something I could do now to lessen my chances of it happening again, but there isn't anything. The disease makes you feel so helpless.

I cannot say enough good things about the care given to me by my doctor. As my estimated March due date rolls closer and closer, I needed to do something to get rid of the feeling of helplessness, so I wrote this article to share awareness of this disease with as many people as I can. I go back to the doctor Monday to finally talk about moving forward with trying again. I am not giving up hope that someday I will be a mother.

June

My name is June Marie. My story begins in the summer of 2011. I started working as a secretary at our church, and I was also asked by our local librarian if I would do story time once a week during the summer. I was honored to be asked to do this job, because my family and I had only been living in this rural town in the upper peninsula of Michigan less than a year. This town made our family feel so welcomed by everyone.

In June I missed my period and felt some of the symptoms of being pregnant. I was worried, scared, and also excited about having another child. My husband and I already were blessed with three children: Kathleen, age sixteen; Noreen, age thirteen; and Erin, age ten. I was now forty-one years old and had always thought that it would be wonderful to start what some people call a "second family." I started thinking how great it would be to finally have a little boy to carry on the family name.

As the month of June went on, I started becoming more and more tired. I would come home after work and lay down on the couch to take a nap. I remember my friend would call me to go for walks, and I would have to push myself to get up and go, even though I would feel great afterward. I didn't think anything was wrong; it was only that I wasn't young as I had once been.

On July 13, I started bleeding. I thought at the time I was starting my period because I was stressed out about my new job and the summer reading programs. The bleeding stopped and started again. On July 15, my morning sickness started. Then it got worse. I had a very hard time eating anything. I went to my brother-in-law's house on July 31 for a family reunion. It was a very exciting time for my husband's family. On Sunday after church we all headed to Detroit for a Tigers baseball game. At the time I was very hormonal; I even yelled at my sister-in-law, which I usually do not do. I also still felt nauseated the whole time. At the ball park I remember walking up the steps to our seat; I was out of breath, and my heart raced. I didn't say anything to my husband, because I wanted to stay for the game. Afterward we stopped to eat at Subway, and all I ate was a banana.

The next day I finally called the doctor's office and was told that my first appointment was scheduled for August 19. On August 15 I called to see if I could get in sooner. I explained to the receptionist what my symptoms were, and that same day the midwife called and asked me if I would come in to get a blood test. When the doctor got the blood test back, the midwife called me to let me know that yes, I was pregnant; however, my hCG level was really high. She scheduled me for an ultrasound for seven o'clock in the morning on Thursday, August 18, the day before my doctor's appointment. This day would change everything for me and my family.

That appointment time worked out great for me, because I could get back to work by nine. At the ultrasound, the technician didn't say anything. I had a feeling it wasn't good. Right at the end, she turned on my heartbeat and my husband looked at me as though he had heard a baby's heartbeat. He had a face like any father would when they find out they're having another baby. He had a wonderful smile. However, I knew the heartbeat I heard was mine and not a baby's, because it was not fast enough. I didn't tell him what I thought. I didn't want to disappoint him.

I got back to work on time, and just before I came home for lunch I decided type my symptoms into WebMD.com. The search result came up with molar pregnancy. It scared me to see that there was no baby and that it could lead to cancer. I quickly got off the website; I didn't want to believe that I could have this condition. When I came home for lunch at one o'clock, I got a call from the doctor's office. The midwife said that I had had what was called a molar pregnancy and that I had to have surgery. I remember her asking if I ever heard of a molar pregnancy, and I answered "yes, it's not a baby."

I started to cry. I couldn't talk to the midwife because I was so upset. I finally calmed down and thanked her for everything she had done, for getting me in for a blood test and the ultrasound. I had so many fears of surgery. Part of it was because I had just started reading a book, *Heaven Is For Real*, the day before. The midwife asked if I had children and if I needed to make arrangements for them, and she explained that I needed to get a bag ready because I would be admitted to the hospital today. She also told me that she would call me in about an hour to let me know exactly where I needed to go and my room number. When I got off the phone, I got into the car and drove to the office where my husband was working to tell him what was going on. He stopped what he was doing and came home. Then the midwife called with my room number and instructions for where to check in. She told me that I needed to be there at four o'clock and that the doctor would see us around five. I had my girls pack me a bag for the hospital because I was so upset, but I told them that they should still go to cross-country practice. All they knew was that I didn't have a baby inside of me and was going to the hospital.

I did not know what to think. On my way to the hospital, I called my mother and explained what was going on. Then we stopped at my in-laws' house to tell them that I was on my way to the hospital and that I needed to have surgery.

After we got to my room, my husband called his sister, Alice, who was a social worker at the hospital. The doctor, a gynecologist, came right at five o'clock. He seemed nervous as he came into the room. He took a chair and moved it to the center of the room. My husband was sitting at the edge of the hospital bed and I was sitting in a chair against the wall under the television. My sister-in-law was sitting in the chair directly facing me. The doctor introduced himself, and in his hand he had a notebook. He started asking about my medical history, how many pregnancies I had had, and so on. At that point of time I had had three cesarean sections, my right ovary removed when I had my first child in 1995 due to a tumor, and a miscarriage in 2008. The doctor told us our options and explained that the molar pregnancy could attack other organs of my body and lead to cancer.

I was scheduled for a computed tomography (CT) scan for later that evening. After he left, a nurse named Diane came in and asked me to get dressed in a gown, and then she put an intravenous line into me. The laboratory technician came in at the same time to draw blood. I was told I couldn't eat dinner until I was done with my scan and had to drink two bottles of some apple-flavored gritty drink, which I thought for sure I would throw up (I didn't). I had to drink the first within an hour, and then the other. By eight o'clock a guy came into the room with a wheelchair to take me for my CT scan and chest X-ray. At this time my husband left to our daughters so I could see them when I was done with my tests. I returned back to my room at nine, and I was happy to see my three girls. Now I had to wait through the night and the next day to find out what was going on.

That night was such a long night. A nurse came in to ask if I wanted something to eat. I said a ham sandwich sounded good, but when it came I couldn't eat more than two bites. I didn't sleep at all that night. Around four-thirty in the morning, I heard the nurse come into my room to set up the bed for an outpatient who was having surgery. She arrived around five o'clock with her family. I didn't see her, because the curtain was pulled, but we exchanged a few words. She was wheeled out of the room by six o'clock. The doctor came in to see me around seven-thirty. He asked if I had decided what procedure I wanted. I told him I had decided to have a hysterectomy. He said he wanted me to think about it and to talk it over with my husband; he would to talk to us again later when he received the results from the CT scan. Then he examined me. Just before he left, he squeezed my foot and told me I would be okay. My husband came in to see me just before eight o'clock. He stayed with me, and we talked. Around ten he left to see his dad and said that he would be back before one o'clock.

The doctor came and told us he had some good news: there was no sign of cancer. Boy, were we happy! We still needed to decide if we wanted more kids or to have a hysterectomy, however. It was clear to us that a hysterectomy was our best option. With a hysterectomy I had less than a thirteen percent chance of cancer. That word *cancer* was so frightening that I wanted to come out of this healthy so I could be there for my three girls. I was told that the earliest I would be able to have surgery was Monday and that I would need to stay in the hospital all weekend.

After the doctor's visit my husband left to get the girls from daily mass. Around two in the afternoon my priest came to visit me, and after he left, my mother-in-law came to visit. Then at five o'clock the priest from the local parish came to visit.

I was so tired; I tried to get a nap but couldn't. Friday night in the hospital I ended up taking a sleeping pill, which really seemed to help. I was able to sleep from ten that night until three in the morning. Throughout the day Saturday the nurses would come and check on me. Some would ask what a complete molar pregnancy was, and I did not mind telling them, because I knew this was very rare. They would ask if I was in pain, and I would say no; I was just nauseated and unable to eat.

I kept myself busy by reading my book. At times I had to stop reading because I knew I was getting closer to my surgery. The doctor who was on duty came in to check on me in the morning. She said that she had only seen one case like mine when she was doing her residency and that she couldn't believe that I had not come in sooner after all the morning sickness. Later on Saturday, around eight o'clock, the nurses came to let me know they were going to move me to my own room. That was fun; I didn't have to get out of bed as they wheeled me down the hallway.

Sunday morning my priest came to give me communion, and then my mother-in-law returned just as he was getting ready to leave. After noon I was only allowed to have liquids. In the afternoon, around three, I received a visit from some good friends, and then around dinnertime my priest came to give me the sacrament of the sick. That was very special; I remember him praying for the doctors and nurses who would be a part of my surgery. After midnight that night I was not allowed to have any food or water.

During these three days I wasn't given any medication, just an intravenous line for fluids. The day of the surgery I remember getting up early in the morning and getting onto the stretcher to be wheeled down to sedation. In the hallway I said goodbye to my daughters; my husband was able to come into the sedation room with me. The girls went upstairs to my room to wait with their aunt. Later, the nurses had the girls go into the waiting room with my husband to wait until I returned. My procedure was scheduled for nine that morning, and I was in surgery for three hours.

I remember waking up around four in the afternoon. I was in my room, and my legs were in straps and being shaken by some kind of machine. I remember asking the nurses to stop it, and they did. There seemed to be two or three nurses in my room. I remember being in pain and very tired. The next day the doctor came to look at my stitches, and I remember him saying that they had had to take out my left ovary. I ended up having a bilateral incision, which made it hard to get out of bed. Oh, how it hurt to get out of bed! I felt so weak that I had to use my arms to lift myself up to a sitting position. The nurses help me get out of bed and asked me if I was ready to go for a walk.

"Remember, today is better than yesterday," the nurse said as I was walking. I thought that was ironic, because yesterday I had had no pain while walking. The next day, Tuesday, when I took a walk around the hospital floor I remembered those words, and I have continued to remind myself every day, even to this day.

Later that morning, I was given a shot of methotrexate. I was very scared, because I wanted to know what the effects would be. I got very upset, but fortunately I received a visitor from our church who was able to comfort me even though I didn't know her. When I had gone into the hospital my church had put me on their prayer chain, and she was one of many people in my community who came to see me or sent me flowers and cards. This lady was like an angel at the time. She was able to have the nurse get me the information I needed about methotrexate.

On Wednesday morning when the doctor came to see me he told me that my hCG level had been 1.2 million and that it already had dropped by half. Then he asked if I was ready to go home, and of course I said yes! I was finally released from the hospital on Wednesday night.

The ride home from the hospital was awful. Every little bump on the road hurt my stomach. It was hard to sleep at night; I had seven to ten pillows on my bed. In the morning when I took a shower, it was hard to raise my legs over the bathtub. I had to have my sixteen-year-old daughter help me. I felt like a burden. I didn't want her to have to deal with what I was going through.

On Thursday evening my sister-in-law was kind enough to bring us dinner. I ate little bites because I still felt nauseous from both the molar pregnancy and the methotrexate. My husband stayed home that night and didn't go to the first football game of the season. I ended up throwing up and couldn't move fast enough to get to the bathroom. When I was throwing up my stomach would hurt. I worried that I would rip open my stitches. After I cleaned myself up I returned to the living room and sat down on the couch. I then noticed my legs and feet had started to swell. I started to panic and had my daughter get me the information about methotrexate.

I was taking five hundred milligrams of hydrocodone/APAP every four to six hours. It took me two weeks to finally sleep with only two pillows. On Sunday, August 28, I didn't go to church because I knew I wouldn't be able to sit for an hour on the hard wooden pews. However, later that afternoon I went to the church picnic. It felt great to get out and visit, although I had to sit on a pillow. My appetite was still not very good; I only ate a few pieces of fruit, a hot dog without the bun, and a few sticks of celery. On August 29 I went to see my doctor and was asked how my pain was. I told the nurse that if I sat still, I had no pain, and that I had stopped taking hydrocodone because it was keeping me up at night. My doctor said he could give me something else, but I told him that I didn't need anything.

That Friday I went to the high school football game. However, I was unable to go into the stands because I couldn't walk very far, and I knew I would be unable to sit on the bleachers. I couldn't even wear my clothes because my stomach was so bruised and swollen. I ended up staying in my in-laws' van to watch most of the game, and then walked in to watch when there was just about four minutes left.

Before my surgery, my husband and I had signed up to help out at the county fair's Right to Life booth on September 3. When that day came, my husband asked me to go with him and just sit for an hour. As I was removing the sheets off the display, however, I saw the different stages of a pregnancy and had a meltdown. I started to cry so hard, because I knew that I no longer had a uterus and didn't have a baby inside of me. My husband told me it would be all right, and eventually I pulled myself together. I couldn't talk to most of the people who came to the booth. My doctor and his family ended up stopping by while we were there; I was so grateful for everything he had done for me and my family, and I finally got the chance to tell his wife.

On my next visit, September 6, my hCG level went from 15,000 to 1,563. I felt so good that day because now I was reading the book *My Molar Pregnancy* and had found the support group on Facebook. I didn't want to have to go through chemotherapy. During this week I was now getting my strength back and was able to go the football game that Friday. I was already back at work, even though the priest told me that I didn't need to be there, but I needed to get the bills paid and order supplies for the church and office.

I went every Monday to get my blood drawn. On September 14, my level was at 532. I was starting to feel better about myself and now my strength was increasing every day. On September 21, my husband came with me to the doctor; my level was at 241. During this week I felt my breasts getting smaller. It was a weird experience, because they say you're not pregnant with a molar yet I still had all the signs of it. September 26, my level was 137. On October 3 it was 113, and I remember not being very happy because it hadn't gone down as far as I had wanted. On October 10 my hCG level was 63, and on October 17 it was at 49.73. On October 25 it was down only to 41.86; that made me nervous until my doctor reminded me that as long as it dropped ten percent I didn't have to worry.

The next day, October 26, was a bad day. After my shower I started to think about how I now had a scar and that would always have it to remind me of what I had been through. I started to think about the Ciderfest at my brother-in-law's the next weekend and how in 2008 I had had a miscarriage when I was at their house. I didn't know if my emotions were from the molar pregnancy or if I was now menopausal.

On October 31, my level was down to 27.11. In subsequent weeks it dropped to 21.07, 13.45, 8.6, and then finally "negative" at 2.3. I called the doctor on November 29 to see if I could start going monthly for testing, and he said I had to wait three more weeks. My tests for those three weeks remained negative, and at my last weekly blood draw on December 19 I went to see my doctor to wish him a Merry Christmas. I brought him a gift, because he made me and my husband feel as though we really mattered and were not just a number. It was a very heartfelt moment.

The spirit of Christmas was definitely felt in our home that year. On the Holy day of the Solemnity of Mary, I decided to be the lector at mass. I practiced the reading and felt very confident in myself. I did great until I got to the second reading. I was reading from the letter from Saint Paul to the Galatians. As I was reading, I came to the line "God sent his Son" and when I saw the next words, "Born of a woman," I stopped and started to cry. I knew I couldn't stop reading, however, so I pulled myself together and continued. It was hard to imagine that I now couldn't have any more children. Then I heard my priest give his homily; he said it was a new year and that we must look onward. We can't change the past. He was right; I needed to focus on my children and the future.

Around April, I finally got the courage to attend a group called Silent Hearts. I had received the information about the group in the hospital, but I had thought at the time that they could never understand, since what had been inside me had never been a baby. When I finally went to the support group, however, I realized it was good for me to be able to talk with someone about what I had been through. Even though I technically had not had a miscarriage, I felt as though I could relate to what they had been through and could finally talk about my feelings.

June was my last and final monthly draw. On Sunday, June 24, my husband and I learned that my husband's sister-in-law was three months pregnant. I remember telling my mother-in-law how happy I was for her, but then I got angry and somewhat emotional. I remember thinking, "What if she doesn't have a healthy baby? What if she goes through what I went through?" When I got home I went to my bedroom and cried, because all those feelings were revisited.

On June 29, I received the call from my doctor's office that I did not have to go back for any more tests. I was officially done. It was an exciting time. I felt so good that I had been able to overcome this. As the months went on, I saw my husband's sister-in-law's belly getting bigger, and it reminded me that there are struggles in life, some we have no control over, and that it is all in God's hands. God has a purpose for every one of us. As I write this, my husband's sister-in-law has delivered a healthy eight-pound, ten-ounce baby girl.

The birth of this baby girl has marked the happy but emotional end to this chapter in my life.

Karey

I always knew I wanted two kids, about two years apart. I didn't care if they were two girls or two boys or one of each; I just wanted two children who were close in age. I also knew that the father of my children would be Steve, the man I met when I went away to college at Rutgers University in 1994. We married in August 2000, when I was twenty-five years old. After finishing graduate school and working for a few years, we had our first child. Evan was born October 22, 2003. He was wonderful and perfectly healthy, every parent's dream. A year and a half later, in July 2005, we knew we were ready to try for our next baby. Just like the first time, I was fortunate enough to conceive right away. I felt so lucky because I knew how challenging it was for some parents to conceive.

By eight weeks, I was feeling just awful, tired and sick. I couldn't remember it being so bad when I was pregnant with Evan. The ultrasound at that time showed a normal fetus with a perfect heartbeat and everything else seemingly normal, except for the actual size of my uterus. My gynecologist explained that it was unusually large for how far along in my pregnancy I was. Usually, he said, your uterus would only be that big at that point if you were carrying twins. However, he wasn't worried; he said I should just come back in three weeks for a follow-up ultrasound. I remember for those three weeks I continued to be extremely nauseated, much more so than my first pregnancy. However, it was the dead of summer, and I figured no two pregnancies were going to be exactly alike anyway.

On September 22, at eleven weeks, I went in for my follow-up ultrasound. I wasn't worried that something was wrong, but I expected that two little heartbeats would show up on the screen, considering the previous size of my uterus and the fact that I already was starting to show a little. I would love two babies just the same, I knew, but I also knew how hard it was to take care of ONE little baby, let alone two. The ultrasound seemed to take an eternity. Finally the ultrasound technician spoke.

"I'm so sorry. There is no heart beat in the fetus." I remember staring at the ceiling and blinking over and over again.

"Okay," I said. "I just knew I felt too sick for it to be normal." I didn't cry; I was too shocked. She said some other things I do not remember, and then asked if wanted to call anyone. When she left the room, I called Steve. He was driving home from work, and I told him everything the technician had said.

"Oh my God, do you want me to come there? I will come right there if you need me," he said. I told him no, I would be fine and would see him when I got home. Then they had me wait in one of the examining rooms. I remember the look of concern on the doctor's face when he came in. It was a look I would get to know well. After offering his sympathies, we discussed my options. I decided I was not going to wait to have a "natural" miscarriage. I was going in for a D&C tomorrow. I felt so sick and I just wanted it to be over.

The next day, while my mother-in-law watched my son, I had a D&C. I remember being upset but logical as ever, as is my nature, and thinking, *Okay, this is very common, it has happened to my own mother, and in three months we will try again.* It's hard to lose a baby at all, especially at eleven weeks. You really start to get attached. Even still, I was strong and thought everything would be okay in a few months. After the D&C, the doctor told me everything had gone well, except for the fact that I had bled profusely during the procedure, and he had almost had to give me an emergency blood transfusion. I was discharged shortly thereafter and scheduled my six-week follow-up appointment to make sure everything was healing up normally.

I remember that that look of concern was on his face again after he finished examining me six weeks later.

"What?" I demanded.

"Okay," the doctor explained, "your uterus is still enlarged. That shouldn't be the case six weeks later." So he rushed me into the ultrasound room next door. The technician did the scan and wouldn't tell me a thing, but the concentration on her face told me there was SOMETHING not normal about what she was seeing. After I returned to the examination room, the doctor told me what was going on.

"There is a mass in your uterus. I don't know what it is or what has caused it, but that is why your uterus is still enlarged. Whatever it is, it has to come out immediately."

The second D&C was scheduled for the next morning. It was October, and Evan had just had his second birthday. My mother-in-law gladly took him for the day, and I found myself on my back in a hospital gown for the second time in six weeks. I couldn't imagine what the mass could be and was hoping my doctor would enlighten me. Unfortunately, he did just that. As I waited with my husband and in intravenous line in my arm, my doctor came to my bedside with a much worse look upon his face that I had ever seen before. I saw fear.

"Karey, I did a lot of research last night and studied the results from your last D&C," he told me. "You have had something called a molar pregnancy." I remember staring at him blankly. "It means the cells from the pregnancy have caused you to have a cancerous-like mass attach to your uterus, and it has grown two inches wide already in six weeks. It's completely curable by chemotherapy if it hasn't spread to other parts of your body yet, like your chest and brain. There will be no way for you to safely conceive again until one year after your body is free from the mass."

I couldn't believe he was telling me this at my bedside moments before surgery. I looked at my husband, who appeared every bit as shocked and confused as I was. I have to look back and laugh at myself for what I said next, considering a doctor had just told me I had a cancerous mass and was going to need chemotherapy. I realize now I was in denial about the seriousness of the situation.

"What do you mean I have to wait a year to get pregnant? I am not waiting a year! My kids will be so far apart in age!"

He patiently explained if I were to get pregnant, there would be no way to tell if the mass had returned. I was speechless and defeated. Then it got even better. The doctor left and came back quickly with a paper in his hand.

"Karey, when we performed the D&C last time, I had a really hard time getting you to stop bleeding. Now I realize why. There is a good chance that will happen again. I need you to sign this paper, which states that you give me permission to perform a hysterectomy if I cannot stop the bleeding."

I actually laughed at him.

"Are you kidding me? There is no way I am signing that paper! No way. I am not meant to be the mother of one child, and Evan was *not* meant to be an only child. Forget it." I looked at Steve and saw he had gone completely white. The doctor saw my panic starting to rise, and he decided he needed reinforcements. He pulled Steve aside to talk to him. They returned a few moments later, one on each side of me.

"Listen," he said, holding my left hand and speaking to me with a genuine compassion and empathy that is rarely seen in doctors. "I will not let you bleed to death on my table. If that happens, who will be the mother to your two-year-old at home?" I huffed at him, because it was a low blow. Then Steve took my right hand.

"I promise you we will adopt a baby if we have to," he told me. "We can't lose you." I loved him more in that moment than I thought possible. I knew I had lost the argument. "Fine," I grumbled, "I will sign the paper, but don't you dare take my uterus out!"

It's hard to put into words the terror I was feeling the last few moments in the operating room before they put me under. I was going to be completely unconscious and had to trust these people not to take away my ability to have another baby. I did not know what reality I would wake up to. The last thing I remember before the anesthesia took me under was staring at my doctor by the foot of the bed.

"Don't do it," I pleaded again.

"I won't," he answered, but I could tell he was only hoping. It was a much longer surgery than my first D&C, about two and a half hours. He had to be as thorough as possible in the removal of the mole. When I woke up, I was actually crying. I think my horrible fear that I would wake up without my uterus had stayed with me even when I was under anesthesia. It was the strangest thing, and I still can't explain it, but my commotion caused several nurses and the doctor to gather around me. I knew where I was immediately and locked eyes with my doctor. "Is everything okay?" I asked him. He nodded yes. I closed my eyes and cried some more.

The next couple of days were a whirlwind of stress and worry. Although I was thrilled that I hadn't had to have a hysterectomy, we couldn't help but face the fact that the molar cells could have spread throughout my body. My doctor's office made the appointments for my computed tomography (CT) scan and chest X-ray so that I could get them done immediately. I realized much later that if the molar pregnancy diagnosis had not been missed initially, the mass would never have had a chance to grow, and I would have gone straight into chemotherapy. I could have tried to point fingers at my doctor, but he had treated me with such compassion throughout the process, I couldn't think of it. Luckily, all of my x-rays came back negative, so no bad cells had spread to any other parts of my body.

I was referred to the Cancer Institute of New Jersey, where I became a patient of another doctor, an oncologist for women. The first time I was sitting in his waiting room, I still could not believe this was happening to me. Cancer from a pregnancy? It was unheard of. He explained to us about the hCG levels and how they rise astronomically high during a molar pregnancy. He also explained how they would be the marker to measure if my body was free of the molar pregnancy completely. I then understood why I had been so sick and why my uterus had been big enough for twins when there was only one fetus in there. Because my diagnosis had been missed for so long and the mass had had to be surgically removed, the doctor gave me a choice on waiting on the chemo. He explained that, in rare cases, the mole could be completely removed and no further treatment would be necessary. We would still have to wait for one year past the hCG returning to normal to try to conceive.

As impatient as I was to get past the waiting period, I didn't want to get chemo yet if I didn't have to. Who would? So I took the blood test to compare my hCG levels with the ones prior to the mass removal. It was Thanksgiving Eve, and Steve and I were up late preparing food for the next day because we were hosting. My phone rang at eleven o'clock. "Who in the world could be calling me this late?" I wondered. It was the doctor.

"Hi Karey. I just got done with surgery and I saw your blood results have come back. I thought you would like to know before the holiday that your hCG levels have dropped significantly. Now, don't get your hopes up just yet; I told you this rarely happens. But I am okay with taking this week by week, as long as they keep dropping, if you want to. Or we could start the chemo if you don't want to drag it out."

I couldn't help but feel ecstatic. Of course I didn't want chemo yet! Despite my impatience, I decided to wait it out. Over the next four weeks leading up to Christmas, my levels continued to drop. I went to the laboratory every Monday and waited anxiously for the results. Besides the waiting, one of the hardest parts of this time was explaining my situation to other people. No one had heard of a molar pregnancy or could comprehend getting a cancerous-like disease from pregnancy. I printed a brief informational blurb from the Internet about molar pregnancy and starting carrying it around in my purse. That way, if I did not feel like explaining what it was, I would just show the paper to whoever asked. Many people had figured out that I was pregnant just by looking at me before, and now that I wasn't pregnant anymore, I owed them all explanations. It seemed as though no one except my mom and older sister could understand my frustration and fear of having to wait. The fear, of course, was that I was now more likely to have another molar pregnancy. It was constantly in the back of my mind. The frustration of how far apart in age my children would be, God willing, was of little importance to anyone I tried to express it to.

"Just be grateful you have Evan," they would say. What else could they say, really? They were right, and they all meant well. I was grateful for Evan. Every single day when I sat on the floor to play with him, I made sure I appreciated the extra time we were having together because of the circumstances. Yet it still hurt, and I feared that Evan's future brother or sister would be so much younger than he was. I feared they would never bond or have fun playing together. I wanted a sibling experience for my own children like I had had when I was little. I knew there was nothing I could do about my situation but slowly and painfully accept my new reality. I learned then that life rarely goes as planned, a lesson I have carried forward into my life today.

It was just about Christmas 2005 when my levels made it to zero. The year-long wait had officially begun, and I had never had to have chemo, for which I am eternally grateful. Every Monday Evan and I went to the laboratory, and every Friday I called the doctor's office to hear the nurse tell me everything was still okay with my results. My older sister, Lisa, and my mom also checked in with me regularly to make sure the results were okay. They knew how hard everything had been and still was for me. A friend who had gotten pregnant the same time as I had called me in April to tell me she had delivered her baby girl. I was sincerely happy for her, but I remember hanging up the phone and crying hysterically. I should have been delivering my baby then too, not having weekly blood draws and being a patient at the Cancer Institute. There were many moments like that during that year. I am so grateful for the night I found the MyMolarPregnancy.com support group on Yahoo while I was browsing the Internet. This was before Facebook, and I had never really been one to participate in online chat rooms before, but I developed a routine of looking over the forum on most nights after I had put Evan to bed. These people were just like me and knew exactly how I felt. The stories were different but all essentially the same. All of the feelings I had: the initial shock and confusion, sadness, anger, frustration, and fear. They all knew just how I felt, and it became a great source of comfort to me and truly helped me get through the long months of blood tests and waiting.

In November 2006, my year finally was almost over. Walking in the front doors of The Cancer Institute, we were elated that all that was standing between us and the go-ahead from the doctor was one last physical examination and one more month of good blood tests. After he examined me, the doctor declared what we had been waiting for: we were free to being trying to conceive the next month! We got in the car to go home, and I looked at my husband.

"There is no way I'm waiting one more month," I told him. He laughed and said he knew I was going to say that. Steve and I couldn't believe our luck when I got pregnant again right away, and my due date was set for September 1, 2007. That was two years past my initial diagnosis. My gynecologist knew my concerns for having a second molar pregnancy were valid, and I had regular ultrasounds for the first trimester so we could watch everything closely. When I made it to the second trimester, my fears that had haunted me were finally lifted, and the rest of the pregnancy was smooth sailing.

We didn't find out the sex of the baby, but we were sure it was another boy. I was also huge, my stomach measuring bigger than when I had had Evan. We figured that that was a definite sign it was a boy, and we were so excited. The doctor agreed to move the due date up a couple of weeks, and my planned cesarean section was scheduled for August 22. At twelve forty-five that day our baby was finally born, and we couldn't believe it when they told us she was a beautiful girl! I never forget looking at my husband at that moment, our eyes filled with tears. I knew what we were both thinking; it became suddenly and perfectly clear that SHE had been the reason we had had to wait all that time. For her…we had had to wait for her. Our sweet Avary Grace.

My children are now nine and five years old. Avary is in kindergarten. What has been wonderful and ironic for the past five years is how much I have come to appreciate the four years between them. I was able to spend so much time with them individually because of their ages, and I know that would have been compromised if they were closer together in age. Also, when Avary was born, Evan was nearly four and was such a wonderful big brother; he was able to understand the needs his baby sister had and was never jealous. He was and still is her favorite source of entertainment. No one can crack her up the way Evan does. Evan also has been able to teach her things like math and reading that I would never have attempted because of her age, but he always wants to share with her what he learns in school. He makes up most of their games, and she will play along with almost anything he wants. In short, they play together and enjoy each other just as much as they would have had they been closer in age, maybe even better. Steve and I never stop wondering how we got so lucky to have the beautiful family we have. The fact that we endured something very difficult to have it makes it all the more special.

A few months ago, Avary told me that Evan was her "BBF: Best Brother Forever." I knew there was not a happier mother on the planet than me at that moment.

Kayla

My molar pregnancy journey began in 2008. That was the year that everything changed—my life, what I believed about myself and others, all of my expectations and hopes for the future. My husband and I began trying to conceive in early January. We fell pregnant on our second try. I had dreamed of starting a family since I was a little girl. I grew up the oldest girl of seven children, always playing mommy to my siblings and taking on many responsibilities. My life seemed empty now that I had grown up. I didn't care to travel the world, as many of my friends had wanted to do in place of having children; instead I put my post-degree life on hold in favor of paying off loans so that I would be able to stay at home with the child I hoped to conceive. I had asked my husband if we could start trying a couple of years earlier, but he was not ready then. When he finally expressed interest in trying to conceive, I basically somersaulted onto the bandwagon.

Thus began the excitement—the dreams of a growing belly, decorating a nursery, and rocking a baby to sleep. My anticipation ran away with me, and it was all I could think about. I knew that caring for a child would be a challenge, because I had seen my sisters with their children, but I did not care. I just wanted to be a mom and have a little person to mentor and nourish.

Just shy of seven weeks pregnant, I went to a prenatal checkup. The nurse practitioner found some old blood upon examination, and I was asked to take a blood test to check my hCG level. She also sent me for an emergency ultrasound. Even though it appeared that the pregnancy was a week behind, my hCG levels were rising accordingly. (I later discovered that was a serious clue!) The radiologist concluded that I had a blighted ovum. The possibility of a molar was noted on the report, but it was glossed over and not explained to me at the time. I was so grief stricken that I didn't pry further. They offered me options to terminate the pregnancy, and I chose misoprostol, a pill that could be inserted vaginally. Had I, or the nurse, been educated about molar pregnancies, I definitely would have chosen a D&C. This part of the process later haunted me as I reflected on whether early intervention would have prevented the disease from developing into persistent gestational trophoblastic disease.

When I was told my pregnancy would not progress, my heart sank; all naive, happy feelings around pregnancy and what it could be like vanished. It was a painful moment followed by a painful process of purging into the toilet for weeks what I thought were parts of a baby. Every time I purged, it was as though someone were stabbing me with a thousand knives and ripping my soul from my body. After some time, I gathered myself emotionally and told myself to be rational and logical, that this happens to many other women, and that I was perfectly capable of getting pregnant again—next time, perhaps, with a healthy pregnancy. I resigned myself to keep the life I created in my heart forever and move on, preparing physically and emotionally to try again. Yet I would not stop purging matter. Something did not feel right. I revisited my family doctor, and he assured me that if anything were wrong, such as infection, I'd be in a lot of pain. I left his office feeling somewhat comforted but suspicious.

On May 25 I was home alone (my husband was away), and I woke up in bed in terrible pain. The pain was more intense than what I had experienced after misoprostol, but it was similar. I went to the toilet and purged a lot of blood and matter, much more than I had been used to seeing after the miscarriage. I went to the hospital and was told I may have miscarried twins. I couldn't breathe; I felt like I now had to mourn the loss of two little lives. They ran some blood work and noticed that I still had high hCG, and that was when I finally was taken in for an emergency D&C. It all happened very fast. Before the surgery there was mention of a possible molar pregnancy, and I made the obstetrician explain what that might entail. It was the first time I heard the word chemotherapy associated with the condition. I was completely in shock that a pregnancy could turn into something so horrid. It was a lot to process.

After the surgery, I went through the good old watch and wait period to which all molar women are subjected to with our hCG levels. Eventually mine hit a plateau, and I was told that I needed chemotherapy and would need an X-ray to make sure the tumors had not metastasized. For many of you reading, I don't have to explain that moment…the fear, the anger, the dread, just the complete out-of-body experience. This was happening to me, in my twenties! As a result of a pregnancy! Fortunately, there was no metastasis; I was classified as stage I.

I remember well walking into the oncology clinic for the first time. It got me thinking about how my father's side of the family is riddled with cancer. I had fully expected that cancer would pay me a visit at some point in my life; but I had never expected it would be so early. When I sat in the waiting room looking at all the other patients, however, I developed mixed feelings about my experience. I felt unlucky that I had fallen into the small percentage of women with molars who need chemotherapy, and sad that I had to endure this. Yet I also felt fortunate that my prognosis was great, and I was so confident that I could beat the disease. As for being confident that I was capable of a healthy pregnancy afterward or that I could ever get pregnant again, well, that was another matter.

When treatment began I became a stone lady, ready for battle, rarely ever letting myself crack emotionally. I focused on doing everything in my power to keep my spirits up to beat this illness. I reminded myself daily that I was not the sickest patient and that my disease was curable. Still, there were so many traumatic parts of that process, the most traumatic being the PICC line insertion. The radiologist took three tries to get it in. After the procedure was over, I couldn't move my arm, and my hand began to mottle. The radiologist guessed that he may have nicked my arterial vein. He told me to keep a watch that night in case I started having severe pain, which would mean that I needed to get to the hospital as soon as possible because I could be dying! Awful, awful experience. My husband set the alarm every hour that night. I lost range of motion in my arm because the radiologist had hit some nerves, and it took me six weeks to get it back. The PICC line pain kept me up many nights when the chemo had me so fatigued and I just wanted to sleep. It was a form of torture. The blisters from my allergic reaction were no picnic either. Needless to say, that was one of the worst parts of the chemo experience. I am thankful, however, that it saved the actinomycin-D (Act-D) from potentially burning through the tissue in my arm and saved me from have to have many painful intravenous insertions. The day I got it out (August 25, 2008) was one of the best days of my life!

Act-D knocked the life out of me, causing fatigue, nausea, metal mouth, skin rash, hair loss, aches and pains, heart palpitations, and so on. The steroids may have helped ease the nausea but caused a list of other unpleasant symptoms (thank goodness for Senekot-S!). It took me about four months post-treatment to get my strength back through personal training and physiotherapy and perhaps six months to feel like my old self. I had terrible chemo fog, and to this day my memory has not recovered, although it's much better than it was, considering I could not read and retain anything and would forget what I was saying midsentence.

After treatment, when I knew it was safe, I fell apart emotionally, lying on my hallway floor for hours crying uncontrollably, unable to move. It was a lot to deal with. I eventually returned to work part-time where I had to see, daily, a coworker who was due within a day of me. I felt happy for her but sad for myself. Her ever-expanding bump reminded me of what I had lost. When my due date approached, she had already delivered and brought her baby in for everyone to see. I escaped to the bathroom where I had a panic attack and was too ill to return to work the next day.

This concludes the negative part of my journey. I want whoever is reading this to know how low I got. It's important that you see that I came out of such a horrible experience stronger and more determined than ever, with amazing friends and support, a new lease on life and that I eventually found my happy ending. So please, stay with me to see just how that happened.

Once my due date passed, I started looking more forward than backward. I resolved to stop letting the molar pregnancy experience control my life and to take my power back. My husband and I began talking about waiting for the six-month mark to start trying. I had been told to wait one year, but after doing some research I decided to chance trying earlier. We fell pregnant again after our second try. Every day of that pregnancy — even the bad ones with morning sickness, fatigue, and back pain — I was walking on a cloud. I literally smiled while puking in the toilet. I was so happy to be pregnant; I felt like the luckiest woman in the world. It was magic. It's not that I wasn't scared or that felt the naïve happiness that women who don't have failed pregnancies do; it's just that there was so much healing happening. As each week passed my confidence that I was capable of a healthy pregnancy increased. Each day was a day closer to realizing my dream.

For so long, my entire happiness rested upon me getting pregnant and having that child that I yearned for. In December 2009, I gave birth to my darling Edward, the little man of my dreams. The pregnancy was scary; I was always wondering what would happen, if Edward would be healthy, if I would get cancer again as a result of the pregnancy. On the whole, however, I felt strong and had a deep gut instinct that everything would be fine. In retrospect, I think it was due to me mentally fighting back against the molar experience, refusing to let it take over another pregnancy. Once I was told postpartum that my levels were negative, I left the molar experience behind in the dust. Sure, there were occasional dips where negative memories crept back in, but overall I felt empowered by having survived that.

Having Edward allowed me to let go of the molar experience. I came to the conclusion that had *anything* gone differently, I would not have my perfect little guy. I also made some amazing molar pregnancy friends with whom I am still friends to this day. We went from being in the trenches, sharing stories of falling levels, surgeries, chemotherapy, and depression to sharing pregnancy and labor stories, then stories about mommy anxieties, giggling babies, feeding solids, and the like. As dark as your life may seem now, you have to know that it does not have bearing on how bright your future can be.

This past January, I delivered twins. Henry and Claire are just amazing. It's hard to believe that I went from not knowing if I could ever get pregnant again to having three little bears. So when you think you can't handle another day of tests, waiting, chemo, up-and-down emotions, insensitive comments by people who don't understand, seeing pregnant ladies and new babies everywhere, purging bits, blood work, loneliness, depression, frustration…endure and pick yourself up off the floor. There's a little life (or a few) inside you waiting to be created and depending on you to be strong, believing in your strength when you do not. In my experience, there are very few women who have not gone on to have beautiful postmolar children. For some the road is longer than others, but most of us get there eventually. I hope my story gives you strength and convinces you to stay the course. It's so worth it.

Kristin

My name is Kristin. I was diagnosed with a complete molar pregnancy in June 2012. My story begins in the United Kingdom but ends in the United States.

In early 2011, my husband and I decided to move to London for a few years due to a work obligation with his job. We were excited to be given the opportunity to live abroad and explore Europe at our leisure. We were still newlyweds at the time, and without children, the timing seemed ideal. This also meant that I could leave behind a very stressful career and look for different opportunities. Given that this move was temporary, we decided to delay starting a family until we were scheduled to move back home. However, we also decided to let nature take its course, and if we happened to fall pregnant during our time abroad, we would embrace it.

One year later and still not pregnant, I was rushed to the hospital for an emergency appendectomy. In the back of my mind, I blamed my troublesome appendix on my inability to get pregnant. The following month, and only one day late, I decided to take a home pregnancy test. Sure enough, two pink lines appeared. I was thirty-three years old. If I'm honest, I must say that I immediately panicked. I began to question my ability to be a good mother and how this would affect my care-free European lifestyle. Luckily, we were scheduled to move home in six months, so perhaps the timing was right. Several weeks later, after much daydreaming and sharing the excitement with close friends and family, we began to celebrate our news. I began to feel like a mom.

At first, the pregnancy seemed uneventful. Besides the typical adjustments to our lifestyle, pregnancy seemed easy. I did experience exhaustion and mild nausea, but I considered myself one of the lucky few and envisioned sailing through this pregnancy without major complications. Finally, the day of our much-anticipated twelve-week ultrasound arrived. That morning, I began to feel nervous. I never once questioned whether we would see our baby or hear a heartbeat; instead I feared an increased chance of a developmental disorder, because they were commonly mentioned in all of the pregnancy books I had been reading.

This was my first pregnancy, so I did not know what to expect that morning, but I do remember thinking to myself that it was taking way too long for the ultrasound technician to detect an image of our baby. Seconds felt like eternity. Finally, the technician turned to us and said, "I'm sorry. This pregnancy is not viable. There is no baby." I will never forget those words and my instant reaction of fear and panic. As we began firing questions, the technician explained that instead of a fetus, my body had grown an abnormal mass of cells. Hearing those words made me immediately think of cancer. Losing my baby and now facing the possibility of cancer was too much for me to handle. I have little memory of what happened next, but I know that I spoke to several midwives, signed consent for a D&C scheduled for a few days later, and was handed several brochures on molar pregnancy. I spent the next few days in pure agony. The waiting during those days before my D&C was emotionally horrific, but I believe it allowed me the opportunity to say goodbye to my baby and shift my focus toward my health.

The D&C itself was successful, although I cried the entire day. I recall one of the surgical nurses reminding me to smile, which felt incredibly insensitive given what I had experienced. I am sure she didn't understand what I was going through. This was just one of many insensitive comments said to me by medical professionals as well as friends and family. At that moment, I began to realize how little was actually known about this disease and just how rare it was. This is what ultimately led me to seek counseling and online support groups, for which I am grateful to this day. Once the procedure was over, my husband and I decided to take a week to ourselves. He stayed home from work so we could be alone. This was a very bittersweet time for both of us because it allowed us to escape from reality and lean on each other for comfort and support.

One week later, one of the midwives called to confirm that my pregnancy was indeed a complete molar pregnancy. I would be referred to Charing Cross Hospital to begin biweekly hCG testing. Prior to the D&C, my hCG levels were over 400,000. I knew I had a long way to go before reaching normal levels. I remember feeling very confused about how the testing process would work. Every two weeks I would receive a box in the mail containing two small tubes for collecting blood and urine. However, I would have to return to the prenatal unit at my local hospital for each blood draw. I could not handle sitting among happily pregnant women knowing that I had been one of them just a few weeks earlier.

The initial testing period was probably the hardest for me. During this time I became obsessed with searching the Internet about molar pregnancies and the likelihood of it becoming cancer. I must have asked the women of my support group a million questions about how quickly my numbers should be dropping and for warning signs that this was indeed cancer. Although these women were incredibly helpful, I felt depressed knowing that many of them had developed cancer themselves. Their stories seemed tragic, and I was scared. I couldn't seem to locate a woman in the group whose numbers dropped within eight weeks and who went on to conceive a healthy baby three to six months later. I also began to hate my body. The small bump that I had cradled in the early weeks of pregnancy became foreign to me. I began to feel that the body that I once relied on and seemed strong had let me down.

Although my family was extremely supportive of me and I missed them desperately, I was grateful that we were still living abroad. I felt that this time away allowed me to truly get in touch with my feelings and grieve privately without the constant reminders and the news of which of my friends were having babies. It would have been impossible for me to share in their joy. I was jealous. I did not understand why this had happened to me. Knowing how rare this disease was made me even angrier. I began to compare the odds of this happening to those of being struck by lightning or hit by a bus; at times I considered anything else tragic to be a blessing compared with what I was experiencing. I felt that my world was crashing down and that things could not possibly get much worse. When people would tell me to look at the bright side, I refused and became extremely bitter. In fact, I would completely shut down when people tried to remind me that there had never been a baby to begin with and that at least I was able to conceive. The fact that there was never a baby made it even worse. I felt cheated that I had never gotten to experience the warmth of a baby inside of me. Still, I allowed myself to grieve as if there had been. It had been real enough to me. I began to feel as though I had failed at being a mother and had let my husband down. I became angry and depressed.

Several weeks later, after yet another routine blood test, I received the dreaded call from Charing Cross. My numbers were rapidly increasing, which meant that the cells were continuing to grow. I had jumped from approximately 7,000 to almost 18,000. It was now cancer. Now, I know this may sound absolutely crazy, but when my numbers began to rise, I actually recall feeling a huge sense of relief. The stress of worrying about my numbers increasing along with grieving the baby had become too much for me to handle. I could finally let go of those feelings and begin focusing on getting myself better. This seemed a lot more productive. Two days later, I was admitted to Charing Cross for one week to begin chemotherapy. My oncologist had me on the United Kingdom's standard 50-mg methotrexate/folic acid regimen. I bled heavily during this first week of treatment and spent much of the week on hospital bed rest.

Once I was discharged, my husband and I used our private insurance to establish private nurse visits to administer my treatment. Our home in London was forty-five minutes away from Charing Cross via public transportation, so I was grateful that I did not have to leave home during the early rounds of treatment. The methotrexate symptoms were really starting to set in at that time. Besides fatigue, I had mouth ulcers and very dry eyes. My worst symptom was pain in my left lung, which made the simple task of coughing or yawning completely unbearable. Luckily, I had a very welcome visit from two of my closest friends from home who came to help me and lift my spirits. I also had the challenge of coordinating our overseas move back home that was scheduled to take place in just a few short weeks. Although it was overwhelming at times, I was happy to have this distraction, which helped me look forward to returning to our home in the United States and finally being reunited with our families.

Another challenge was trying to coordinate my care once we returned to the States. I had grown close to the team at Charing Cross and feared that my care in the United States would fail in comparison. To this day, I feel extremely fortunate to have been at one of the leading hospitals in the world for this condition. With the help of one of the online support groups, I found a woman who was completing treatment at a hospital near our home in New Jersey. She was kind enough to pass along the name of her oncologist, who had agreed to follow the same treatment regimen that I was receiving in London. He even agreed to consult with the Charing Cross team on a regular basis about my care. Finally, the day had come to move back home. As luck would have it, our flight home was scheduled during my third cycle of methotrexate. Charing Cross packed me with several injections of methotrexate so I could complete the current cycle in the United States.

Once we returned home, I completed four more months of chemo. My treatment was administered at The Cancer Center at St. Barnabas in Livingston, NJ. I am extremely thankful to my parents, who drove me to and from each injection. They made the entire experience much easier for me and filled my days with much love and comfort. Their support made every difference to this experience. Although the care I received was very good, it was different from what I had had in London. My new oncologist took a much more conservative approach. He immediately ordered several scans of my lungs, liver, and brain, which is where the cancer was likely to spread. Although I appreciated these precautions, I can't even begin to explain the fear I felt with each scan and pending results. The results of my lung scan showed several nodules on my right lung that may or may not have been a metastasis of the cancer. A scan done in February 2013, one month after my last treatment, came back clear.

By late October 2012, my levels began to hover in the single digits, still above normal. This happened to be during Hurricane Sandy, which of course makes the experience completely unforgettable. I recall receiving yet another dreaded phone call from my oncologist explaining that it was time to switch to a more aggressive form of chemotherapy, which also meant worsening side effects and the possibility of losing my hair. That was my biggest fear, and I refused to believe that this was my fate. I was convinced that if given one more cycle of methotrexate, my numbers would once again begin to drop. I decided to call my oncologist at Charing Cross, who agreed to convince my current oncologist to give this one more shot. Luckily, my instincts were correct and after my next round, my hCG dropped to 5. I was now only a few points away from "normal."

Several days before Thanksgiving, my hCG finally reached 3, or "normal." I had so much to be thankful for. Once again, my oncologist had agreed to follow the Charing Cross standards and administer three additional rounds of chemo to ensure that my hCG levels remained at normal. I took each of these injections with a smile and a huge sense of relief, knowing that the end was near. On January 4, 2013, I had final injection. My parents were with me that day, and we cried as I left the hospital for the last time. Two days later, we celebrated the end of this long journey on my original due date. I thanked our baby for watching over me.

Today, I am five months into my year-long waiting period. Though I still go for routine hCG testing, I am happily enjoying my break from doctor's offices. I carry a lot of pride in my ability to survive this both physically and emotionally. I feel that this has given me a whole new appreciation for my health. Wishing someone health and happiness has an entirely new meaning to me, and when I say it, it comes from my heart. I also have an overwhelming sense of gratitude for our families that have blessed us with so much love and support. I also feel that in life, things happen for a reason and that with every bump in the road, there is a lesson to be learned. For me, that lesson is that I am a lot stronger than I ever gave myself credit for. I am also grateful for a stronger bond with my husband. I never envisioned that we would be dealing with something so serious just a few years into our marriage. Yet after surviving this, I am certain that we can survive anything as long as we are together. Most important, I've learned that it is now my mission in life to become a mother and if that day comes and I am able to finally hold a baby of my own, I will realize that this was all worth it and that I truly have been blessed by a miracle.

Krystal

On April 11, 2010, I took a home pregnancy test and it was positive. This pregnancy was a little earlier than I had planned, as my firstborn was only six months old. I was nervous and scared and felt that I had cheated my daughter out of being the baby. This pregnancy started off badly, with low hCG levels that were not rising as they should. On May 6, 2010, I had my first miscarriage. I was heartbroken and felt guilty for not being happy when I first found out.

On July 23, 2010, I found out I was pregnant again. I was overjoyed. My hCG levels were rising, but my progesterone was low, so I immediately was put on a progesterone supplement. My first doctor's appointment was August 24, 2010. I was eight weeks along and feeling really good about this pregnancy. I went in for an ultrasound, and my doctor's first question was, "Did you get a positive pregnancy test?" At that moment my heart dropped into my stomach, and my stomach felt like it was in my throat. After I told him that I had, he looked at my chart and studied the monitor a little more closely. I couldn't look at it. I could barely breathe. Then the words came out of his mouth. "Krystal, I think you have a molar pregnancy." I was sent directly over to the hospital for a second opinion and scheduled to return to my doctor that same day at four o'clock for a follow-up. My husband had returned to work after my first appointment that morning, and I felt so alone. I went home and cried for the couple of hours in between appointments. I knew in my heart that it was going to be the end of this pregnancy. At four I returned to the doctor's office. I could see it on his face that he had been correct in his earlier prognosis. He told me it was confirmed that I was having a molar pregnancy and that I needed to have a D&C as soon as possible. I was scheduled for a D&C at seven o'clock the following morning. My doctor sent me home with one of his medical books to read up on molar pregnancy so I could understand a little better about what was going on. I searched on the Internet but did not learn any more than I had already known when I started. I was amazed at how little information was available on the subject.

My husband is a very loving man, but he does not handle sad situations well. He also sucks when it comes to providing comfort for a miscarriage in any form. He doesn't believe life starts with conception. When I got a positive pregnancy test, I was having a baby. I had imagined what he or she would look like. I had already painted the room and begun to get decorating ideas. I had an entire future planned for this little tiny ball of cells. My husband told me "Well, at least it wasn't a baby." I have never felt so sick in my life. Here was this man I have known and loved for seven years, the father of my child telling me that the baby we conceived wasn't really a baby. I went and took a shower and cried until the water ran cold and then cried a little more. I felt broken. What had I done to deserve this? Why was my body so stupid that it couldn't realize I wasn't even pregnant with a real baby?

August 25, 2010, at seven in the morning, I went in for my D&C. I cried the whole time I was in pre-op. The D&C went as planned and had no complications. The rest of the day, I just felt hollow. The day before my D&C my hCG had been 207,451. I returned to my doctor for a follow-up on August 31, 2010, and my hCG was down to 4,400. I was told I had had a complete molar pregnancy, meaning there never was a baby. He said that I needed to wait six months before trying again so we could be sure that the mole did not come back. After the specifics, he asked how I was doing and feeling. I told him I had not slept in a week, so he gave me a prescription for Ambien. I didn't tell him that I was depressed. I was too ashamed that I was grieving for a baby that did not exist. I was to return a week later.

The Ambien helped the first night; I slept like a rock. The second night was not so good, I had hallucinations. I saw a little girl on her bike fall into a well, and I couldn't save her. I believe that was my body trying to warn me that I couldn't save myself, that I needed help. I wish now I would have gone to my doctor about my depression, talked to a counselor or something.

On September 8, 2010, my daughter's first birthday, I returned for another follow-up. My hCG was 393. I was told I would need to go for blood draws every week until I reached zero. The following week, September 15, my hCG was 45. On September 23 I went in for my last follow-up appointment. My hCG was 12, and I was told I would have to wait a year to try to conceive. I was so mad that he had changed it from six months to a year, but I didn't ask questions. I just wanted to be done with this whole mess. I didn't want to argue with my doctor about it.

Four weeks later my hCG reached zero. During my wait to zero I had found a support group on BabyCenter for women who had had molar pregnancies. The only reason that I didn't have a complete mental breakdown was the ladies on that board. My husband was no help when it came to support, and if he saw me crying he would give me a look as though I were pathetic. I know he didn't do it on purpose, and he may not have even known he was doing it. During the next few months, I pushed him away. The ladies on that board gave me a place to go to feel normal. They have a special place in my heart, and I so very thankful to have found them.

I made the decision to only wait six months before trying to conceive again. I did not come to this decision easily. I did research and made sure I was confident in going against my doctor's instructions. I started temping my cycles and went full-blown crazy woman. I took the fun out of having a baby. March 29, 2011, while on a much-needed vacation to Las Vegas with my husband, I got a positive pregnancy test. That was the happiest I had been in a very long time, but the happiness was replaced with fear the moment we got home. On April 4 I called my doctor and scheduled an appointment. I went for my first hCG draw that day and every two days after. My first draw was 339, my second was 750, my third was 1,986 and my fourth and final was 4,962. I went for my first appointment April 19. I have never been so nervous and terrified in my life, even after everything I had been through that year.

My doctor lectured me on getting pregnant so soon after my molar, and I broke down. I lost it right there on the table. I couldn't look at him or at the ultrasound monitor. I was embarrassed about being lectured like a toddler, and when I told him that I had done my research he made a comment about the Internet being a doctor. I was irritated, so I stared at the wall until he started to talk about my baby. I was five weeks pregnant and everything looked good. No sign of a recurrent molar. I returned two weeks later for a second ultrasound and saw a perfect little baby with a beautiful heartbeat. I had an appointment every two weeks until I was out of the first trimester.

I thought I should have felt "normal" at that point, but I didn't. I allowed fear to take over my pregnancy and did not want to bond with a baby that wasn't going to go home with me. I cried before every appointment for nine months. I had never gotten over my molar pregnancy, and I allowed it to take over my life. I was so consumed with numbers and weeks and months that I forgot to breathe. I just wanted a baby at any cost. Not only did this affect me but it also took its toll on my marriage. I didn't know how to open up to people anymore. I felt like a failure to my husband, to my daughter, and to the precious tiny human who was growing inside of me.

My pregnancy flew by somewhat uneventful. I was scheduled to be induced with my son on December 2, 2011. Even going into the hospital that morning I was terrified that something would happen to my baby. My labor was fairly easy. After my water broke, however, the baby's heart rate started to drop with every contraction. It turned out that the umbilical cord was wrapped around his neck twice. I never told anyone this, but I was sure that he would die during labor. Fortunately he was born perfectly healthy. He was a few months old before he and I really bonded with each other, however. Having a miscarriage and then a molar pregnancy had taken the joy out of my life. It took all the innocence out of being pregnant. I had lived on autopilot for that year.

It has now been three years since I traveled down that road. I am currently pregnant with our third and final child. I am still very early in my pregnancy, but I am at a place where I am not full of fear every single minute of every single day. I have finally accepted that I have no control over what happens. I am enjoying this pregnancy the best I can, because once it is over, it's over. There are no redos, no second chances. I have been dealt the hand I have, and it is up to me to make the best of it.

I am a stronger person because of my past. My marriage is stronger because of the struggles we went through. I have come out on the other side with knowledge of things I never knew existed. I have friends all over the world whom I have never met in person, yet we have all traveled the same stretch of road. We are connected by a story we never chose to be a part of. I am so very thankful that they were there to walk it with me. If I could give advice to someone going through a molar pregnancy it would be to live your life. Grieve for what could have been, but don't let it consume you. You will come out on the other side.

Lisa

Our daughter was turning one, it was early December 2011, and life was great. My husband Stuart and I had just pulled off a fantastic party to celebrate this amazing year for sixty of our family and friends, and I was exhausted. My period had not come yet, but I had not been that regular; I had had only had three cycles thanks to the wonders of breastfeeding. I put my feet up after our daughter went to bed, and my husband was snoring. An intense sense of urgency came over me in a wave. "What if I'm pregnant?" Being impulsive, I drove to the shops for a home pregnancy test and took it as soon as I got home. Pregnant! How amazing! We had not been trying but were not doing anything to prevent it either. This was the best news considering how much we were enjoying new parenthood and the struggles we had had in the past to conceive.

The coming weeks were a beautiful time. My husband was extremely proud of his roaring fertility, and there were new plans on our horizon in the lead-up to Christmas. When I shared the fantastic news with my mother, which we did straight away, she was not surprised. She claimed that she had left Aimee's birthday party and confided to Dad that she had thought I looked different and wouldn't be surprised if I was pregnant.

Mere days before Christmas we were booked in for our first scan. The technician was quiet, and there was no real sense of chitchat to calm our nerves as we waited to hear what she saw. The only words we got from her for a full five minutes were, "Unusual, no gestational sac." We waited, almost too frightened to look at each other. With Aimee we had had early ultrasounds, and we were puzzled by what we could see now on the screen, just a mottled grey snowstorm appearance in my uterus. We left full of apprehension, but all we had been told was that perhaps it was simply too early to see anything clearly. We made an appointment for another ten days' time.

New Year's Eve rolled around and, despite the cloud hanging over our heads, at least we had a party to go to with lots of great friends. Then BAM! Everyone is pregnant. Two of our friends announced that they were expecting babies, and both were due the same week as us: August 17, 2012. With a bit of coaxing from Stuart we decided to share that we believed we were pregnant too but had not had a great first scan. One of the girls who had just announced said the same thing had happened to her, but when she went back a week later everything was fine. This news brought us hope, and there was then much nattering and planning throughout the night about all of the new babies we would be welcoming in the year 2012.

The date of our second scan arrived, and we were firmly and quickly informed, "I'm sorry to tell you, I have no idea exactly what I am looking at. The only thing I can tell you with any certainty is that it is not a viable pregnancy." It sounded so clinical, so matter-of-fact when I felt like that was the furthest thing from the truth. My husband had not been able to contemplate that this was what we would hear, and we were both shell shocked. I swear I almost had a nervous breakdown.

My heart felt empty, yet I managed to sob openly, not caring who would see me or even where I was anymore. When I could breathe and speak, I rang my obstetrician, who let us go straight to her office. She called through to the fetal medicine department at the Canberra Hospital, and they had a specialist up from Sydney for the day who would not be back for another fortnight, so we were rushed into a slot. It was terrible sitting in the poky waiting room with the walls lined with heavily pregnant women who were expecting and complication free.

Again we heard the words, "It's not a viable pregnancy." The specialist sonographer did, however, add that it did not look to be a classic molar pregnancy. She commented about not seeing a bunch of grey grapes; the ultrasound was more just a snowstorm to her trained eyes.

We then ferried ourselves back across town, where the obstetrician advised that we do nothing and wait for a natural miscarriage. This was heart-wrenching news, knowing that something was growing inside me that was useless tissue that I had to hold onto. Seeing no spotting, I was in denial about what the experts were telling me. Never before in my life had I felt so torn between my plans for the future and my reality. Time passed slowly and I still had no bleeding, so a D&C was scheduled for January 12. We were told that some tissue from the procedure would be sent off to the laboratory for testing. The results would likely take ten days because they had to grow the tissue in the lab to continue looking at it.

The diagnosis actually came back within four days; it was indeed a complete molar pregnancy. Strangely this news was a relief for my husband Stuart; he was able to logically conclude that we had not in fact ever lost a baby. I suppose since he had not had pregnancy symptoms—swollen breasts, morning sickness, and extreme fatigue—he was unable to compare this pregnancy with our last successful one. This difference of views has continued to this day to cause fights between us, because to me, we did in fact lose a baby. I certainly know we conceived one.

A week passed, and one of my pregnant friends suffered a miscarriage. She rang me knowing I was the person who would understand most. We shared our despair over how unfair it was to hurt so much. I felt a sense of guilt that was happy to have someone to share my grief with in an uncensored way. There were times over the following months when I believed my luck was far worse than hers, but I tried to vent this online through the My Molar Pregnancy Support Group instead.

After my D&C I began blood draws each week to monitor that my hCG levels were dropping down to where they needed to be, which was less than 5. Blood drawn on the day of my D&C showed that these levels were at 210,000. A week after, I was at 8,000, and I began a steady decline until I hit around 1,000 eight weeks later. I then had two "insignificant" rises. It was at this stage that I was first referred to an oncologist to look at beginning chemotherapy.

I decided to participate in Australia's World's Greatest Shave, which is a fundraiser to provide money for leukemia treatment. At this stage I was going through some severe "survivor's guilt"; I knew that my persistent trophoblastic disease was 99 percent curable going down my treatment path, and although I was upset by it all, even worse was thinking about being diagnosed with something that did not have such great patient outcomes. Sitting in the oncology ward at my local public hospital with people who were terminally ill with their cancers was by far one of the most traumatic parts of my whole experience with a molar pregnancy. Raising $9,000 for the cause left me, for the first time in months, with a positive feeling.

At my first visit with my oncologist she recommended we start a course of methotrexate then and there. I was totally unprepared for this news and told her it was not possible because I was still breastfeeding and would need at least four days to wean my fifteen-month-old. Over those next days I relished Aimee's morning feeds. I was torn because I had wanted to continue feeding and felt a sense of being in the passenger's seat of my own life.

The following Monday I commenced my first round of chemotherapy. I was given intramuscular shots of methotrexate, 10 mg, on days one, three, five, and seven, with folic acid given on days two, four, six, and eight. These were followed by a week off medication. This continued for six cycles from March until May 2013. My blood draws were each fortnight, going from over 1,000 to 663, 148, 56, 9.7, 3.8, 1.7, and finally less than 1. When I saw the oncologist, she told me I would now have to wait twelve months until I could be cleared to try to conceive again. My wonderful girlfriends planned a night out and surprised me with a massage voucher and money kit to spend on drinks and taxis. However, I was tired; this had been the worst part of my treatment cycle and I still had one last needle to endure in the morning.

A few of my friends announced pregnancies over the next few months while my blood was being checked monthly. They each knew my journey, so they called me privately on the phone to let me know. I was flattered they thought of protecting my feelings and allowed me the chance to rehearse being excited for them before they announced to other friends at parties.

After five months of tracking my blood results and having no other treatment, I forgot to have one test. Although this hormone is a pregnancy one, it is also the tumor marker my oncologist was using to ensure I was not relapsing into gestational trophoblastic disease. When I called for the results of the next test before Christmas, my numbers are at 385 (they have been under one for the past six months), and upon hearing this there is no doubt in my mind that I am pregnant. My husband thought exactly the same way and was rather chuffed with his supreme fertility, seeing as we were not trying.

There was a sense of dread sitting heavily on my chest. I was excited to be pregnant but was still waiting for medical confirmation that this would be a safe pregnancy. We knew very little about the side effects of falling pregnant six months after my chemotherapy treatment, and I was unclear as to my risk of another molar pregnancy. I needed some advice, so I booked an early ultrasound at six weeks. The second of January felt so far away.

We went for our ultrasound and saw a little heartbeat. I was so pleased to see that perfectly round black gestational sac on the screen. My pregnancy suddenly became a little more real. I had just turned thirty-five years old, so I supposed I was medically considered a geriatric pregnant mother. I cried when I learned my doctor couldn't look after us because she would be on holiday around the time we were due. We went back to our general practitioner for advice on a public birth, and he said we sounded most comfortable with an obstetrician and gave us a referral to see another doctor.

As I write this I am thirty weeks pregnant and looking forward to the birth of a healthy little boy.

Lori

"I am so sorry" are not the words you want to hear at your first ultrasound scan with your first pregnancy. The pregnancy up until then had seemed normal. The pink line showed up on the home test, and I was blessed not to have nausea for the first nine and a half weeks. Then nausea came on with a vengeance until that eleven-week scan, but other than that I had had all normal pregnancy symptoms and no indication that anything was wrong. Little did we realize that this was the beginning of a long and confusing journey. As we arrived at the gynecologist's office, we were grinning from ear to ear. This was our first pregnancy, conceived on our first month of trying, and here we were, beyond our wildest dreams, about to see our baby on screen for the first time!

The gynecologist looked and indicated that she was not able to see much so she had to do an internal scan. That was when it all fell apart. Instead of a fetus, the screen showed only a grayish, snowy mass. She indicated she was 95 percent sure it was a molar pregnancy but would only be able to confirm this on pathology and would need to do a D&C as soon as possible. She spoke about monitoring, explained that the tissue was precancerous but unlikely to develop into anything worse, and told us that a second D&C could be necessary if the tissue was persistent. She also mentioned chemotherapy. It was such a shock that I didn't register much of what she said at the time. We contacted my parents, who were overseas at the time, and at that point I burst into tears at the realization that I wasn't going to have my baby in my arms in the next few months after all. We went home and started researching what a molar pregnancy was.

I had had what is known as a complete molar pregnancy. My blood levels were taken at the time of the D&C (August 2008) and were 300,000. The following week they had dropped to 3,300 and it looked as though it wasn't going to be too bad to deal with. Then the added blow came that we were not allowed to try to conceive again for a year because the new pregnancy could mask the tissue regrowth. Great, so not only did I have this freakish condition, but now I had to wait twelve months to try again! I had to have my levels monitored weekly and started to feel like a pin cushion. My levels dropped again over the next week to 2,300 and then went back up to 3,600 so I had to have another D&C (mid-September 2008).

Over the next few weeks they dropped down into the early hundreds. Then the monitoring continued and continued, with my levels dropping bit by bit, until the day they leveled off and hit a plateau at 187. (A plateau is defined as a decrease of less than 10 percent of your hormone levels consecutively over a period of three weeks) The next shock came: I was to be referred to an oncologist because the tissue was now considered to be persistent. I went to the oncologist, who did a CT scan and an MRI scan and diagnosed me with low-risk persistent gestational trophoblastic disease. WHAT?? He recommended that I start chemotherapy as soon as the medical aid (medical insurance) gave consent. Up until that point I had been fairly composed, but when I heard I had to start chemo, my world came tumbling down. I needed professional help to deal with the way this was all turning out. I found an amazing therapist (who had never heard of a molar pregnancy either), and we started on my emotional healing. We dealt with scores of different issues including the pregnancy loss and what I would do if my hair fell out from the chemo (e.g., buy a wig or wear a scarf). Somehow discussing everything rationally with someone who wasn't emotionally connected to the process in any way was very grounding, and it helped me to see a clear, practical path of how to navigate the whole situation.

I began the chemo in early November 2008 with a daily infusion for five days every three to four weeks. On alternate days I also received antinausea medication. Every time I went into the oncology center and saw the other patients there (most of them gauntly thin with no hair), I was reminded of how "lucky" I was to have my condition and not theirs. It's weird how you put things into perspective and rationalize what you are feeling, but I really did feel lucky being me, in that outpatient clinic.

We had booked an overseas trip to London and Israel in December to see family. The oncologist worked my treatment around our trip so we were still able to go. I was fortunate that the chemo had worked very well and I had only two rounds of treatment to get my levels back to normal. I began to bleed about two weeks after my first chemo and panicked. I went to the gynecologist who sent me for a blood test. I was overjoyed to learn that my levels were only 65, a great sign. She said my body was confused and the bleeding was probably a "fake period." It was a step in the right direction. As it so happens, I got my period four weeks to the day after that bleeding and it continued every four weeks to the day for most of the following year. I never imagined I would be so relieved and thankful to have a period, but it meant that my body was okay and that it was working normally. I still am thankful every month when my period arrives, because it reminds me that I am healthy.

I went back for my second round of chemo (which was right before our trip overseas), and the oncologist agreed that he wouldn't test my levels until we returned from the holiday to make sure I had a relaxing trip. We had the most wonderful holiday, and when I came back I was tested and my levels were less than 5 (which my doctor considered negative)!! I had to have two further rounds of precautionary treatment to make sure that the tissue had resolved.

During my treatment I had a number of different side effects: my hair thinned, I got mouth sores, and I had nausea (which worsened as the chemo days progressed) and constipation. I was lucky enough to work for a very supportive company at the time and took off the five days of treatment and went back to work the Monday after. The day of my first treatment I went out for lunch with my family and felt great, but by two days later I wasn't feeling so well anymore and every day would come home from treatment and sleep the rest of the day away. I spent the days of my treatment in a cotton-wool-like daze and had very poor short-term memory. I am a planner who likes details, so I wrote myself copious "to do" lists to make sure I didn't forget anything important. The last day of my last chemo cycle was ironically the worst day in terms of side effects, but I was so happy to be done with chemo that I did not care. It was Friday, the 13th of February 2009, just four weeks away from what was supposed to have been my due date for the pregnancy. To this day, I consider Friday the 13th a lucky day.

Another side effect from the treatment was that my immune system was low so I managed to catch whatever illnesses were going around at the time. This continued a few months after treatment as well. I caught a cold two months after treatment that lasted for about six weeks, and I coughed so much from it that I dislocated one of my rib joints!

The oncologist and the gynecologist agreed I should wait twelve months from the last treatment to start trying to conceive again. I was so frustrated and at that point "just wanted to try for a baby" that I contacted a molar pregnancy expert in America who confirmed my doctor's recommendations. Thus, we waited. The first half of the twelve months was extremely difficult because two of my closest friends had just had their babies (we were all due within three months of each other), and everywhere I turned there were bumps, babies, and toddlers. It was devastating. I found amazing support groups online and still keep in touch with the ladies from these different groups; they helped me to deal with what happened in so many different ways. Unfortunately most of the ladies I found were overseas, but I did find one in South Africa, and we still meet up once in a while. It took me a few months to share my story with family and friends, but I found that as I started talking and explaining what I was going through and had been through, I felt stronger and stronger emotionally.

The next six months were much easier, and I kept myself busy with work and recreational activities. I also found myself looking for security in my religion and friends, and I started a regular prayer group where we said psalms both for ourselves and for others needing prayers. I also started attending a ritual bath (Mikve) designed for the rite of purification and attended weekly synagogue services during which time I reconnected spiritually with God.

We were cleared to try again in February 2010, and we were back at the gynecologist's office in early May after a positive home pregnancy test. The gynecologist sent me for blood tests to check that my hormone levels were rising appropriately, and when we walked back into her office, she was grinning from ear to ear because everything looked great. Postmolar pregnancies are normally followed very carefully in the beginning to ensure that it is indeed a new pregnancy and not regrowth of tissue, so we were nervous but excited. On our first scan she couldn't find a heartbeat yet but told us to come back the following week. The second time, there it was: a perfect heartbeat! The doctor was amazed and elated and commented on what a textbook pregnancy I was having this time around.

As the pregnancy progressed and everything remained normal, I felt less and less anxious. The anxiety never truly left, however, and I used to pray the night before each doctor's appointment that everything was okay. The molar pregnancy had taken away any pregnancy innocence I had ever had; however, it helped me realize how lucky I was to have a healthy pregnancy this time. I embraced every bit of morning sickness, every ache and pain, every late-night toilet trip, all the reflux, stretch marks, et cetera, because they reminded me how blessed we were with this pregnancy.

I had regular scans to make sure the pregnancy was progressing normally and delivered our beautiful little girl in December 2010. My placenta was sent off for testing to make sure it was clear of molar cells, and I had a six-week postpregnancy blood test to check the same. I never imagined after what I had gone through that I would have a healthy, perfect child. I struggled at the time to understand why I was going through the molar pregnancy, but at some point in my treatment I found meaning in what had happened to me. For me, it was a wake up call that I was living on autopilot, taking life too seriously, working like a demon and not really enjoying life. The experience forced me to slow down and reassess things. I sometimes wish that God could have taught me that lesson in a less traumatic way, but I know that would not have worked for me. I also know that if I had not gone through this, I wouldn't have my precious daughter.

We gave our baby two very special names to recognize the experience and the growth that came out of it—her first name means "G-d has healed" to acknowledge both my physical healing as well as my and my husband's emotional healing that He guided us through. Her middle name means "life or living one" in testament to the living, breathing person that she is (as opposed to the mass of cells I carried in the molar pregnancy) and to reflect how blessed and grateful we are that we were able to bring a new life into this world.

Our daughter is now three and a half, and we are very thankful that her little brother is on his way. There is no doubt that she brings abundant joy and sunshine to us, and all those around us. I often watch her in wonder and can't believe that this little person calls me "Mommy," a word I wasn't sure I would ever hear. All babies are miracles of nature, this little girl (and her brother, due in October) are ours.

Misty

I am twenty-seven years old, I have an amazing husband and a five-year-old little girl who is my sun and moon. I live in a small town in Oklahoma. I have always been pretty healthy, minor health issues. I am a normal girl, so I never expected how much my life would change in a year's time, how I would have to rebuild my life and myself. I didn't plan on submitting for this book, but a good friend told me "Never be ashamed of your story, it could help someone." The My Molar Pregnancy Support Group has become a part of my life; although we have never met, the women there are my friends, and I have to check on everyone daily. They are my people.

April 2012, after a year of trying, I found out I was pregnant. I had had symptoms early on, but I thought I wanted it so badly that my body and mind were just making it happen. I took one test and looked at it quickly. When it said I was not pregnant, I just sat it on my dresser and went on with my day. Later, however, when cleaning up, I was about to throw the test away when I saw it was positive. It had been longer than ten minutes by then, however, so I didn't think there was much to it. Yet when my period didn't come I waited another five days and then got up at five in the morning to take another test. I didn't want my husband to know until I knew; trying had been hard on him, and I didn't want to get his hopes up. This time it again was positive! I didn't believe it, I took still another one, and it was positive too. I woke my husband to tell him. We both were so happy. We took announcement photos to give out on Mother's Day. I went to the doctor to get my tests all started. I hoped to get an ultrasound before Mother's Day because I wanted to include copies with our announcements. We made an appointment for the Wednesday after Mother's Day and figured that was close enough. We gave our mothers each a cute announcement, and they were happy and excited by the news. We told our four-year-old daughter as well, and she was excited to become a big sister.

Wednesday came, and we excitedly went to our appointment to see our baby. I was eight weeks and a day. I sat on the table and unbuttoned my pants. As I waited for the ultrasound technician to find the heartbeat, I got really nervous. I think I knew something was wrong before we walked into the room. This pregnancy had been completely different from my first pregnancy, but I did not want to think about it because then it would be real. I never thought what happened next would ever happen to me, or that it was even possible. The tech asked if I was sure of my dates, and I was. He decided to do a vaginal ultrasound instead, so I undressed, and he returned with the doctor's assistant to observe. I kept telling myself it was because he had to have a woman in the room. Again they couldn't find anything. I had a placenta and a sac but no fetal pole and no baby. The assistant took my daughter out of the room, and the doctor came in. He looked at the ultrasound and said "I've never seen anything like this; in med school there was something like this. It's called a molar pregnancy. I know you need a D&C scheduled but I'd like to send you to someone who has seen this before."

That's when my life changed. The assistant printed me some paperwork that explained what a molar pregnancy was. Then I was sent for the first of many blood tests. I could not stop crying; everyone looked at me with pity at the hospital. I couldn't speak. The person who took my insurance gave me a whole box of tissues. She was very nice but had no idea why I was there. When they finally called me back to get my blood taken, they asked why I was crying. I just handed them the papers I had been given. She read the first line and told me she was very sorry and hoped that the test would show nothing. I knew it wouldn't; my empty womb was forever burned into my memory. I cried the whole way home. I had to tell my step-mom what had happened so that she would watch my daughter. Again I couldn't say the words, so I just handed her the papers and kept crying. She told everyone while I cried. They kept saying they were sorry and that they loved me anyway. I spent the night crying; my husband called everyone for me and made my appointments. A friend came and got my daughter so my husband and I could process the situation. My husband was amazing through everything. He hardly cried; he just kept making phone calls and making sure I was okay. I had to call my stepdad and my mom to ask them to keep my daughter during all of my appointments. I tried to explain to them what had happened but they didn't understand. They just believed that it was a false pregnancy. I think the hardest person to tell was my daughter. How are you supposed to explain to a four-year-old something adults can barely understand? My husband and I told her that the baby was sick so it had had to go live in heaven. She asked some questions and seemed okay with our answers.

The nearest oncologist and hospital I was referred to was an hour away. I went that Friday to have another ultrasound. It looked the same, and it felt the same to see it and know. My oncologist, whom I had not yet met, called and told us if I started bleeding or anything to call her and she would call me right back. I don't think I understood how serious this was. Monday I met my oncologist for the first time. She was a quiet, sweet lady and never made me feel like this was something she could not handle. I felt an instant trust. After hours of paperwork, questions, and an exam, she sent me to the hospital where I was going to have my surgery. The hospital treated me wonderfully; they made sure we understood everything and that both my husband and I were taken care of. That night of course I could have no food or drink after midnight.

Tuesday, May 22, 2012, my husband and I woke up at six to be at the hospital by eight. I was so scared; I know he was scared too. He kept telling me how much he loved me and that everything was going to be okay. It was nine by the time they got me back to my room; the night before there had been a shooting at tailgate party for our NBA (National Basketball Association) team, so the operating rooms were busy. The nurses didn't understand what a molar pregnancy was; they had to do a pregnancy test before the surgery. One nurse had to ask someone when the test came back positive. Once things got started my memory starts to blur; I remember being moved from my room to the operating room, and as they put the mask on me I started to cry again. My doctor came over and promised me everything would be fine and she would do her best. She held my hand until everything went black.

Again everything is very fuzzy as I woke up. I was in pain, and they kept giving me morphine. The tubes had scratched my throat when they removed them. I remember someone looking for my husband. My doctor told us that she barely had to scrape my uterus, that everything had gone perfectly. I had to take a birth control shot and then was sent home around one in the afternoon with antinausea medicine and painkillers. The morphine stayed with me longer than I would have liked; I slept the whole way home, and when I got home I slept until about 6:00 p.m. A wonderful friend came over to sit with me while my husband went to get my medications. She also made us dinner and stayed with me the next day.

I was lucky my numbers dropped from about 200,000 to 1,200 the first week after the surgery. I was told I had had a complete molar pregnancy. I had weekly blood tests for six weeks. The levels kept dropping, but I still did not feel like I thought I should. My body did not like the birth control shot I had been given, and I had had previous issues with birth control pills. The shot mixed with the hormones, and my grieving made me crazy. I convinced my doctor to let me go off birth control so I could try to get control of myself and start moving on. I began to search for something, anything to help me with what I was feeling. My husband and I spent hours together Googling everything. I eventually found a book called *My Molar Pregnancy*, and after "Liking" it on Facebook, I found the support group. I met other women who knew everything I was feeling and had been through this and made it to the other side. For the first time since I found out I was not having a baby, I felt less alone.

Once I made it to "normal" I felt like I was safer, even though I still had to get monthly blood tests. It became a new way of life for my family. We hung out in outpatient care waiting to get my blood work done; we waited on phone calls; during the summer we even went to the movies and made the trips into special days for our daughter. I tried to make life as normal as possible for her. I put grieving on a shelf; it wasn't fair to her for me to upset her life. I was very depressed for months, and I was angry at my body for betraying me. It was a lot to process and work through. My due date had been December 23, 2012, and that was a very hard day. I was supposed to be having a baby, not grieving a baby.

I spent the rest of the year grieving, crying a ton, and talking with the support group and my friends. On June 6, 2013 I was "cleared," which meant I was done with doctor visits, tests, and waiting on phone calls. My doctor left me a voicemail that I have listened to a dozen times. I finally told more than just the people who were close to me. I now tell everyone that I have two children: one holds my hand, and one holds my heart. This has been the hardest thing we have ever been through. I will always grieve for what should have been, what could have been, and what will never be. I will never be the same.

Nurse

I remember having this talk with a coworker/old sorority sister of mine once. She and I weren't close; we were just having a casual conversation at our orientation for a new job, and she mentioned that she never wanted to have kids. It was surprising to me. Sure, I know people choose not to have kids, but I had never witnessed anyone say it. I come from families where all of my aunts and uncles are married with kids. I don't think of myself as naïve either, but I simply couldn't relate at all. It isn't that I thought less of her or judged her in any way; I just couldn't understand how someone could be so sure of themselves on such a matter. I wondered if she would regret her decision when she was older. Since I was very small there had been nothing I wanted more than to one day get married and have kids. It had never been a question for me.

On November 24, 2009 I gave birth to my first child, our daughter Camille. The pregnancy went fine; it was just a long nine months and with lots of nausea in the beginning. My labor story, depending on who tells it, was a little more dramatic. I thought it was quite comical, even a day after. As one nurse put it to me: "Well, the first thing is you had to be induced, and the other problem is you're a nurse." I was induced a week after my delivery date, starting with Cervidil cream at around ten o'clock the night I arrived at the hospital. I had some cramping and contractions for the next twelve hours because of the cream, but my cervix remained undilated. I had not slept in two or three days. The next nurse who came on duty made it her goal for the day to get me to sleep. They started Pitocin, but she hardly titrated it up at all in her twelve hours. I asked for a pain pill around noon that day, and she gave me some old drug that she said would make me feel hot. She chuckled and told me to take it and pretend I was at the beach. I really just wanted Tylenol or ibuprofen, but they don't give any of those so I took what I was offered. She had convinced me this would help with the discomfort and maybe help me sleep.

I had a few family members in my room, and the next thing I knew I was burning up as though the building were on fire. I began taking all my clothes off and kicked my family out of the room. I cursed and laughed to my husband about how terribly hot it was and how had I known what the nurse meant, I probably never would have taken the pain pill. I laid back down but never fell asleep. When my next nurse came in I was twenty-four hours into hospitalization and still my cervix had not dilated at all! It was unbelievable when I look back, but it makes me laugh. This nurse and the doctor cranked up the Pitocin first thing that morning, and away we went. I probably didn't actually qualify as active labor until maybe three the next morning. I was able to have a nap after they broke my water and placed the epidural. I finally delivered my daughter around seven o'clock on the morning of November 24.

I was exhausted at this point from not sleeping, the long hospital stay, and labor. My doctor came in for my episiotomy, and all I could do was close my eyes and try to relax. He stitched it even though the placenta had not released itself yet. Then, discouraged, the doctor at some point realizes my placenta isn't going to come out on its own so he reached up to yank it out. This kind of freaked me out. I am a nurse, and I remembered learning about the placenta in nursing school. It was not common for the placenta to stay attached. The doctor said it happened once or twice a year for him. The nurse's aide reacted out loud and said, "Okay, so we need to get her in for a D&C, right?" just after he pulled out the placenta. The doctor said no and held pressure to stop the bleeding. I asked him at a follow-up appointment later if I needed to be concerned about this placenta ordeal with another child, and he told me no, and I asked my next gynecologist a few years down the way if I needed to worry and was again told I did not.

It wasn't long before we were able to try to conceive again. I have depression and anxiety and was taking medication, so I had to wait a little for those to get under better control or at least get on safe medications for pregnancy. I had some depression after Camille, but since I had already had a history it is hard to say whether that was postpartum depression or just me being myself again. So, we tried to conceive for four or five months with no pregnancy and multiple episodes where I was sure I was pregnant. We finally started logging everything and trying on fertile days, and within one month I was pregnant. I was overly excited, as I am very much that type that gets a little too excited over things. Camille had been telling people I was pregnant for about nine months before that because she wanted to be a big sister so badly. I knew how special she was and knew she was going to make a great big sister. In fact, I was quite content with my family already, but my husband wanted another child and Camille needed to be a big sister. In truth, the thought of caring for myself and two children really frightened me a little.

Anyhow, we made Christmas cards announcing Camille would be a big sister and then announced to the family and Camille on Christmas. I was nine weeks pregnant at the time. Camille got a bag that said big sister and had a binky and bottle and stuff inside. She was thrilled. On the airplane home from a nice Christmas in Denver I noticed I had some bright red bleeding, and it continued for several hours. I called the doctor and a nurse line and bawled to my husband for an hour. I had read in one of my pregnancy books about an incompetent cervix and that was the hope I clung to, because it was the only thing that fit that seemed fixable. It was the only thing that didn't mean miscarriage. At this point it was just the threat of losing the pregnancy that scared me. I fell asleep for the night.

The next day the doctor told me to drive to the emergency room. Most people would not be able to sleep at a time like that, but I have insomnia (another weird diagnosis), so I always have sleeping pills.

In the emergency room the nurse practitioner came in and told me they suspected a molar pregnancy. At ten weeks along and having had six weeks at least of nausea throughout the day, I was devastated. I looked like I was five months pregnant compared with my first pregnancy. I knew right away what she meant, at least partially. I remembered molar pregnancy from nursing school because it was such a "weird" thing. I said to the nurse, "You mean the one that isn't even a real baby?" She said yes. I bawled out of control for what seemed like hours. A week later I learned my hCG levels were initially 191,000 (December 29, 2012), and my D&C results showed a complete molar pregnancy.

My husband had told my daughter while I was at the hospital, and she had cried to him. She was just over three years old. She was smart, so she knew and understood both the big sister bit and now that there was no baby. She started her own grieving as well. It was a really sad time. My husband came up to drive me home from the D&C, and Camille went to stay with her grandparents. On our way home I called my mom, and she said Camille was dragging around and sad. Mom had asked her if she was worried about her mom, and she had said yes. The next few weeks were rough. Camille would notice babies in restaurants and look at them and ask when she would have a brother or sister. She picked up a magazine from the grocery with pictures of baby twins on it. I could tell she was struggling through it the best she knew how. I was getting notes home every day from her daycare about her not listening or having trouble focusing.

I read a lot about molar pregnancies and cried some. Although I had recognized the condition from nursing school, I hadn't remembered the cancer and chemotherapy or possible hysterectomy part of all this. So I learned a lot from the girls on the Facebook My Molar Pregnancy Support Group and read a lot on my own. I started to imagine the worst right from the beginning and felt like I just wanted to get rid of it and never have to go through it again. I wished I could just get a hysterectomy and forget about it.

I went to work that Wednesday after a few days off work to take it easy. I was very open and honest with the people at work about what was going on because I knew this could be a long and bumpy road and I wanted people to know what I was going through as well as why if I had to miss work in the future. People were so kind. I got flowers from coworkers. One male nurse overheard me discussing it and start telling me about him and his wife and how she had had three or four miscarriages before they figured out what was wrong. I just stood there looking at him with a blank stare. It felt like I didn't say anything. I had to go back and apologize to him days later and explain. I told him I was sorry, I was just still trying to accept what was happening and process it. I explained it was a molar pregnancy, but in his case just as in many others, he didn't know the difference. People hear "miscarriage" and think that is it. I had to have a discussion with my own mother about it as well. She wasn't really saying anything about it at all. I finally asked her if she had looked up molar pregnancy and she said, "Well, no, it just sounds like you had the same thing I had and Sandy your stepsister had." I explained to her that night that it was actually different and told her all about it. She apologized for seeming distant and told me she felt it was pure ignorance on her part.

My follow-up appointment arrived. My hCG levels had dropped to 21,111 within a week. That was a lot. My husband was wowed by this. I still had a bad feeling; I didn't find the news reassuring at all. It was only one test, and I guess I needed to see a trend of them dropping to get my hopes up. I had an episode of bleeding either the day of or day after my follow-up appointment; it came on suddenly and I felt the gush of blood. I monitored it, and after I passed a large clot it subsided and went away. I had some nausea following the D&C, which surprised me, but that too eventually went away.

On January 13, 2012, I was at work and had a second episode of post-D&C bleeding. I had a gush of blood followed by three pad changes in two hours and a large blood clot. This was the second time, so it didn't take me long to call my doctor. I went to the emergency room and was kept overnight and into the next day. They did an ultrasound, a chest X-ray, and a CT scan of my abdomen. Lots of laboratory samples were drawn. My hemoglobin had dropped to 10. My blood pressure was still in the 98–102/58–70s range, which are both low for me but not critically low. My hCG was 32,000 now, up from last blood draw. My doctor scheduled a D&C for the next morning, but cancelled it and asked a female oncologist to see me. Dr. Murray came in prior to my abdominal CT and chest X-ray. She explained they would at least be trying methotrexate on me but maybe other chemotherapy agents depending on the test results. She would give me the first dose in the hospital, and I would get weekly injections afterward at my follow-up appointments.

The nurse called a while later and said the tests had come back and I could go home. I told her it did not make sense that they still had not treated me for my primary problem—the vaginal bleeding. I said the doctor had told me I would be taking at least methotrexate and would be starting the medication here in the hospital prior to leaving. The nurse said she would check into it, but Dr. Murray was in surgery. We waited until about 4:30 p.m., and I found out I would be getting just methotrexate. The nurse finally came in with my shot at about 6:40 that night. She had regular gloves on and when she looked at the methotrexate she said, "Oh, it says chemotherapy." She then had another nurse check it with her. She told me "You have to get this in your bottom; I don't know why." I corrected her and told her the doctor had said it was to be given intramuscularly in my hip. She administered the shot in the wrong spot for a hip injection. It was testing my patience and started making me lose faith in the medical system more than ever. She went on to tell me how she was teaching at a local community college for nurses. This pissed me off more, because young nurses should be taught to always look up medications they're unfamiliar with and the proper administration instructions prior to administering! Intramuscular shots aren't something most nurses do often and it is okay to forget, but you need to look this stuff up prior to giving it. I just prayed I would not have any problems from the incorrect shot site.

I was so ready to go home. I hadn't seen Camille since the prior morning on her way to school, about two whole days. I had been texting my husband asking him to try and keep her up until I got home. I finally left the hospital about eight o'clock and was able to tuck in my daughter and read her some bedtime books. I told my husband we were lucky because years ago I might have just bled to death.

In the hospital while the oncologist was taking my history and asking her assessment questions she had asked about my previous pregnancy and if there had been any problems with it. Then she asked if had been any problems with my labor. I got really quiet and felt a sense of dread and anger. She then said, "I mean, any problems with the placenta?" I thought "Oh God, this is all related!" I knew my experience had been abnormal, and I had been so worried about it even though doctors had told me it was fine. After I told her about my placenta she asked if they had done a D&C afterward. My mother and husband were in the room, and my mother later told me she had wondered if I had put it together. She had picked up on the same thing. It wasn't that I wasn't mad or disappointed in my previous doctor, but I was curious if he had just been lazy not doing the D&C or just uneducated about it. Was the medical research and information just not up to date? All of these new questions and concerns flooded in. It isn't like I want to sue him, I just wanted to know the truth.

I asked my oncologist later about whether my placental issues were related to my molar pregnancy, but she discounted my concern and made me feel better about it. She said she thought it was unlikely that they were related. I was not completely convinced, but she made me accept the fact that although we don't know for sure, it isn't worth worrying about it.

The following are my hCG levels for the weeks that followed:

- 40,000 on 01/21/2013
- 20,784 on 01/28/2013
- 6,800 on 02/04/2013
- 2,440 on 02/11/2013
- 760 on 02/23/2013

I received three doses once I was negative to be aggressive in preventing further growth. The physician says I can try to conceive again in August 2013 if my numbers stay down. She was happy with the clean drop of a curve my labs showed with the methotrexate treatment. I am somewhat apprehensive about pregnancy still. I am worried it could happen again without a doubt.

Sarah & "Grammy"

"These cravings are going to put a damper on my diet!" That was my Facebook posting on April 14, 2011. I was being congratulated for being pregnant, but there was no hidden meaning behind my post. I was truly on a diet and had already lost twelve pounds. I was less than five pounds away from my goal weight, so I made sure everyone knew it was not an announcement. The next day I was awfully moody. We were sitting at the dinner table at my in-laws' house, and my father-in-law flat out told me I was being a witch (although he used a different word). We kind of laughed it off while I asked what was for dessert. My mother-in-law said there was ice cream in the freezer, and my reply was "Nah, I don't want ice cream, I want a big fat piece of cake!" My husband looked at me and asked, "Are you pregnant? You don't even like cake!" I got defensive and yelled back, "Why does everyone keep accusing me of being pregnant? If YOU said you wanted a piece of cake would everyone assume YOU were pregnant?!"

That night I had so many thoughts running through my head. "Maybe I am pregnant. Nah, I can't be. The doctors told me last year that I would need help getting pregnant." My mind was racing. Everyone was accusing me of being pregnant, and I truly did not think I was.

Saturday morning I woke up early. I had a pregnancy test in my drawer, so I decided it would be good just to make sure. So I did it. I peed on a stick and waited. To my absolute surprise, two lines appeared. "Oh NO!" I thought. "They were right. How could this be? So much for not being able to get pregnant! How do I tell my husband? We were not planning for this. We just moved halfway across the country and he hasn't found a job yet." Again, my mind was all over the place. I called my mom, who is my best friend. We are really close, and I needed advice. I had always wanted to have children, but how was I supposed to tell my husband this unexpected news? My mother suggested that I buy a book about fatherhood and give it to him.

I ran to the store to find the perfect book. When I got home I sat on the bed where my husband was still sleeping. He woke up and looked at me as I told him I bought him something. He asked what it was, and with a big smile on my face I told him it was a book. I was laughing uncontrollably because I was so nervous, and I hesitated to give it to him. After a few minutes I closed my eyes and handed the book over. To my surprise he started laughing when he saw the title: *A Father's Almanac.* Through clenched teeth I whispered, "I am glad you find this funny, but this is no joke!" I understood why he thought it was. I mean, for the past few days everyone had been accusing me of being pregnant, so he thought I was just playing a prank on him. I ran and grabbed the stick and handed it over, yelling "NO! Look I am serious!" He questioned what pink meant. "It's not the pink that matters," I told him. "It is the fact that there are two lines! That means I am PREGNANT!" Still in shock, he quietly asked, "But what if I am not a good dad?"

After the shock wore off, we agreed we would wait to tell people until I had it confirmed with the doctor. Since I already had an annual exam scheduled for that same week, I just called the office to tell them my news. On April 22 it was confirmed. Although it was totally unexpected and not planned, we had done it! We had made a baby on our own. We were thrilled. We didn't need help after all! Because I never really had had a regular cycle, we were unsure what to base the due date on. The doctor assumed that I was somewhere around eight weeks pregnant based on the size of my uterus, but I insisted that I had to either be five weeks or more than twelve weeks along because my husband and I had been in two different states eight weeks earlier. With that information, she said, "Well, that means you are either measuring small for twelve weeks or big for five weeks, which could be an indication that you could be having twins." She laughed as though she were half joking and told me that an ultrasound would give us a more accurate due date.

We went home and told everyone! We started with my in-laws with whom we were living at the time. We let them know by telling them we would need to plan on an extra person for Christmas. At first they thought we were telling them that my mom would be joining us from Pennsylvania, but then it dawned on them. My father-in- law's eyes got big and all he could say was, "Really?!" We nodded and shared tears of joy. After all, this was going to be their first grandbaby. We announced the news to the rest of our immediate families, and the word spread like wildfire.

> **Thoughts From Grammy:** It was one of the most exciting days of our lives, in our family. The news that we would have a grandchild in a few months. It was amazing. Our family was ready for this transition. Our sons had both found wonderful, loving life partners whom we adore, so this was the next step in our family, the next generation. My sisters were already grandmothers and talked about all the activities they did with their grandkids. I was waiting for the day my husband and I could do all these fun things too! So the day we got the news, we were thrilled!

On April 26 we went for the ultrasound to double-check how far along I was. It was too early to see much, but they let us know that there was indeed a gestational sac and yolk but no fetal pole. We were told that I was at five weeks, four days, and my due date would be December 23. I was ecstatic! December 23 is my sister's birthday, and I thought how cool it would be to have a niece or nephew born on her birthday. We were scheduled to have another ultrasound in three weeks' time.

May 8 we celebrated my very first Mother's Day. We had a family dinner, and as we prayed over our food my husband's cousin thanked God for all of the mothers, including those who were expecting. That was me! I was the one who was expecting that we were thanking God for! My heart was smiling! I had such overwhelming joy swelling up inside me as I thought about next year's Mother's Day. I would be holding a baby in my arms!

May 17 came and we were headed to the clinic for our very first sneak peek at our little "bean." Anticipation and joy took over my whole being. We were called back by the ultrasound tech, and I laid down on the table. She put the probe on my abdomen, and there it was. A jumping bean appeared on the screen with a little flicker. We saw that tiny heart beating at 161 beats per minute. As old wives' tales go, we smiled at the thought of having a little girl due right around Christmas. We knew that we couldn't really determine the gender based on the heart rate alone, but it was a fun thought!

June 3 I had my first official obstetric appointment. I had to see the nurse practitioner because the doctor was not available. I was not thrilled about seeing her because I remembered her having NO personality when I had gone in for my annual exam. My husband was also with me, and we were both overjoyed. The nurse practitioner did all the routine stuff and used the Doptone to see if we could hear the heartbeat. After a few minutes of running the probe over my abdomen without finding the heartbeat, she had me go to the bathroom to empty my bladder. She assured me that at times a full bladder can block the baby. We tried again, but there was still nothing. At this point I never thought to be concerned, because she assured me that everything was fine and they only start to worry when they can't hear the heart on Doptone at twelve weeks. I was only eleven and a half weeks along at the time, so I just thought it was too early to hear.

For the next four weeks I continued to walk on cloud nine anticipating life with a new baby. I was so anxious to find out if we would be welcoming a boy or girl into our family and hated the thought that I had to wait until twenty weeks to find out the gender. I had my next appointment scheduled for July 6, and this time I made sure I was able to see the actual obstetrician. I called my mom every morning on my way to work, and the morning of my appointment she asked if I would have an ultrasound later that day. I let her know it was just a routine visit and that the only way I would have an ultrasound was if something was wrong. I did not know then how true that statement would prove to be.

My appointment was not until three-thirty that afternoon, and my husband met me at the doctor's office. We were called back to the exam room and answered all the questions the doctor had. It was time for me to lay on the table to use the Doptone to listen for the heartbeat. I was so anxious. This was going to be the first time my husband and I actually got to hear that precious little heart! After five LONG minutes of the doctor probing around in all positions, we still couldn't find the baby. The doctor assured us that there was nothing wrong and that sometimes the baby is laying in a weird position so it is hard to pick up on those monitors. She said she would send us for an ultrasound just to be sure. My heart sank while my earlier statement to my mom clouded my thoughts: "The only way we will have an ultrasound is if something is wrong." I tried to be positive. I smiled at my husband and giddily told him that just maybe we would get to find out the gender of our baby. After all, I was almost at sixteen weeks, and I had read that sometimes you can find out that early.

The receptionist called over to the hospital and they said they could get us in for the ultrasound at four forty-five, which meant we had to leave straight from the office and go to the hospital. My husband and I texted both of our mothers to let them know that we were headed for an ultrasound and to pray that everything was okay.

> **Thoughts From Grammy:** The day was getting closer when we would find out if we were getting a grandson or daughter. Then came the unexpected day when my daughter-in-law had an appointment and sent me a text that said, "We are on the way over to the hospital for an ultrasound, but don't worry. The doctor could not find a heartbeat today, but she said it is pretty normal for being this early. And then she said we may find out today if it is a girl or boy!"

It was hard to get thirty-two ounces of water down in the short ride over to the hospital, but those were my instructions. We didn't wait in the waiting room long before the technician called us back. We went down a dark hallway and into one of the ultrasound rooms. I laid on the table and the tech asked why I was there. I told her that in the office they had been unable to hear the baby's heartbeat but that the doctor had assured me everything was probably just fine. We were there to double check. The tech agreed and turned the monitor toward us eagerly. She put the gel on the probe and moved the wand around my belly. It felt as though I lay there forever, and I had this horrible feeling that something was just not right. A few minutes later the tech turned the screen away from us and continued to move the probe around while typing on the computer. She didn't say a word. All three of us were silent. I took a few deep breaths as the tech turned to look at us with sadness in her eyes and said, "I am sorry, but there is no heartbeat."

Tears flooded my eyes. My husband fell out of his chair, knelt on the floor, and cried into his hands. At that moment, time stood still and I felt all alone. After being ushered to the bathroom to empty my bladder, my husband and I sat on the table and cried while holding each other. About fifteen minutes went by before the radiologist finally came in. He said, "I am sure you already know, but the ultrasound did show fetal demise. Miscarriages happen to one in five pregnancies, so this is really common. Your doctor's office is closed now, but they will probably call you tomorrow and let you know what the next step will be. Most of the time your body will just take care of this on its own, but occasionally some people will need surgery. Just go home and wait for a call tomorrow." He apologized and left the room.

"That's it?!" I screamed in anger, "This is something he sees all the time, but does he not understand that I just lost my baby?!" I was mortified that he considered me some statistic. We left the hospital still in tears. I just did not understand. I thought that when people miscarried there were signs. I thought there was supposed to be bleeding and cramping. I thought there would have been something to let me know there was a problem. I had had nothing. I had felt wonderful for the past sixteen weeks. I had had no complaints, yet my baby no longer had a beating heart. I called my mom, hysterical. She answered the phone chipper like she always did, and all I could blurt out was "My baby is dead!"

We arrived home, and my mother-in-law met us in the driveway. I got out of the car and screamed through tears. She ran over and hugged me as my husband dropped the cup he was holding and ran inside. My mother-in-law and I cried while holding each other for a few minutes before walking into the house. My husband was sitting on the kitchen floor sobbing. My heart was in so much pain. It hurt for me and my loss but also for my husband. I had never seen him so upset, and to think I was afraid to even tell him I was pregnant!

Thoughts From Grammy: The hour after receiving the text about the ultrasound was the longest of my life. I was out in the yard, pacing and praying that all was okay. I heard their car pull into the driveway, and I ran out front. Within minutes, we knew that our baby had already gone to be with Jesus. Our son lay on the driveway crying, and I stood there crying with my daughter-in-law. Soon my husband joined us, and we all stood huddled on the driveway sobbing. All the joy and anticipation suddenly in an instant had turned into a gut-retching pain. The loss for us, our grandchild, and the pain of our children dealing with the loss of their child—it was dreadful.

I spent the rest of the night laying in bed crying and asking questions. I asked over and over, WHY? What had I done wrong? Could I have done something to save my baby? My husband came into the room and said in a soft, caring voice, "I called your mom, she will be here tomorrow. I figured you would want her to be here." I was ANGRY. I was strong. I didn't need her to drop everything and get on a on a plane to come to my rescue. Why the heck would he even think about asking her to come here? But who was I kidding—she was exactly the person I needed to hold me, cry with me, and tell me that everything was going to be okay.

I decided to go to work the next day. I could have taken the day off, but I figured I would probably just sit around and cry all day, so I thought work would help keep me occupied. On my drive there I called my mom like I did every morning. She told me about her travel plans and the flight she had booked. I started to cry, "Mom, I was angry at Andrew for asking you to come to my rescue, but I really could use a hug." I could tell she was smiling when she said, "I know, there is nothing like a mom hug is there? I will see you later on to-night."

I got a call from my doctor late that afternoon. She told me what we already knew: the baby had died. She said that the baby was only measuring at eight weeks although I was nearly sixteen weeks along, and there was no cardiac activity. She said that most likely the baby had been dead for a few weeks and that my body probably would not miscarry on its own. She recommended that I have a D&C, so I was scheduled to have the procedure the next day. Again, I was in shock. "You mean to tell me that I have been carrying a dead baby for a few weeks? How did I not know?" I spent that evening going from being sad to outraged and angry.

The next morning was Friday, and I woke up early because I had to be at the hospital by eight o'clock. My husband and mom took me in, and we were instructed to go to the second floor. As the elevator door opened, I instantly began to cry. There above us was a sign that showed operating room to the left and labor and delivery to the right. "How cruel," I thought. "I was supposed to be going toward the right just five months from now to deliver a healthy baby, and instead I am turning left to have a surgical delivery because there was no heartbeat." I was taken to a preoperative room, and my nurse entered. She asked me what I was there for and I blurted out in tears, "I am here because I lost my baby." Her eyes got really big and she walked out of my room. How insensitive. She knew why I was there. It had to be in my chart. I am sure it said I was there to have a D&C, so why did she have to ask? I was an emotional wreck. It was not supposed to be this way.

A few minutes later the nurse returned and apologized. I guess she was not expecting me to answer the way I did. Her tone changed and she treated me very kindly. I was so nervous to be having surgery. Just two years prior I had had a reaction after surgery and ended up on a ventilator in intensive care. I was terrified I would not be going home after this "quick procedure." The anesthesiologist asked a lot of questions and assured me that they were going to take good care of me and that everything would be just fine.

After my procedure I received a RhoGAM injection because my blood type is O negative. I was told to follow up with my doctor in two weeks, and they discharged me to go home. I cried as they wheeled me through the hospital hallways and out to our car. I never in my life had felt so empty. Never getting the chance to hold my precious baby consumed my thoughts. That day, June 8, Baby Roberts had been born directly into the arms of Jesus.

Although emotionally I had never felt worse, physically I was feeling pretty good when we got home. I needed a few things from the store, including menstrual pads because I had been told I could possibly bleed for up to twelve weeks. My mother and mother-in-law took me to Target. We were goofing off trying to keep our minds off of everything. We went to Chipotle across the street to have lunch. There was a pretty long line, so we stood there discussing my mom's plans to head back to Pennsylvania the next day. I wished she could stay longer, but she wanted to give my husband and I some time to process everything and heal from our loss. She wanted to give us time to be there for each other while we grieved the loss of our baby.

I looked up, and at the front of the line there was a woman who turned around. At the sight of her, tears streamed down my face. She was a very petite woman and right in her midsection was a belly the size of a basketball. I was angry. How dare she stand there in front of me, pregnant, due any day while I was here grieving the loss of my own baby! I was mad at HER for some reason. Like she should have known the pain I was going through. Like it was her fault she was there the same time we were. I was furious that she was pregnant and I no longer was. I questioned why God didn't think I was good enough to have a baby. What made that woman there in Chipotle "worthy" of having a child, while mine was taken away from me?

Later that evening my husband asked me how I felt about having a memorial service for our baby. At first I was shocked. I never would have thought that my husband would be the one suggesting that we call the pastor to see if we could have a service to acknowledge our loss. I questioned if it was okay for us to have a service for a child whom we never met. Miscarriages are such a taboo subject, and no one was supposed to talk about it much less hold a service for the loss. To us, however, that was our first child, even if we never got to meet it. I agreed that maybe it would help bring some closure, and I knew that if he was asking for it, he probably needed it! His mother called the pastor and let her know our tragic news. We all agreed that we would hold the service that Sunday afternoon.

I knew I wanted to do something special at the service. I wanted something to symbolize the precious wings that God had given to our baby and its spirit that lived on. Butterflies floated through my mind, and I knew that a monarch was exactly the symbol I needed. I did some research online and found a woman who had a butterfly farm about four hours from our house. I wrote her an e-mail explaining our situation and asked if I could buy just one butterfly although her website only showed that she sold them in bulk.

The next morning, Saturday, I checked my e-mail as soon as I woke up. To my surprise I had a reply from the butterfly lady. She extended her sympathy and gave me her phone number so we could talk about how I would get the butterfly from her. As we spoke on the phone she told me that she had a worker who would be driving to the fairgrounds just fifteen minutes from my house later that day and that she could send my butterfly with her. She gave me her employee's phone number, and we arranged to meet that afternoon. The employee gave me a hug when we met as she explained understanding what I was going through. She knew what it was like to lose a child and was thankful that she could be there to help us in our situation. I was so amazed of the generosity of two women who had never met me before. They had gone so far out of their way on such short notice so that I could fulfill the need of a symbolic butterfly release.

Before church on Sunday morning we met with the pastor to talk a little bit about the memorial service we would be having later that day. We agreed that the memorial garden would be the perfect place to remember our baby, and she assured us that she knew what to say during the service. We were told that we could do whatever felt right to us, and she was thrilled with the idea of releasing the butterfly into the garden. Our loss was announced to the congregation during the regular church service. Many people gave us their condolences and shared their own stories of loss. Our family spent the next few hours preparing for our baby's service.

We met in the memorial garden at two that afternoon. Twenty-seven family members gathered there with us. The pastor made our loss so real. She let us know that even though we never got to meet him or her, our baby still lived and would always be a part of us. She told me I was still that child's mother and encouraged us all to look forward to the day we would finally get to embrace. She made mention of the fact that we ask lots of questions in times of loss and that we may never understand all of the whys. She acknowledged that it would be hard to see other pregnant women and to see children but encouraged us to embrace the babies around us because every child was a miracle. She validated all of the feelings that I was going through, and I had never even verbalized them to her. I read a poem that I had written to our sweet child, and then my husband and I released the butterfly while the song "Dancing With Angels" played. We all smiled at the sight of the butterfly hanging around the garden, exploring its new surroundings. We had the opportunity to take pictures of the beautiful creature before it sailed on the breeze and into the skies. The service was absolutely beautiful, and I was glad my husband had brought the idea to light. We felt honored to have so many family members there to acknowledge the life of a child who had never breathed our air. The one person who was missing was my mother, but she had already gone back to Pennsylvania.

> **Thoughts From Grammy:** Our son asked if we could have a memorial service, and our pastor said some very comforting words. Our daughter-in-law and son planned a beautiful service with many family members in attendance. That service was to be the beginning of our healing. They released a butterfly at the end of the service, and now that butterfly has become a very meaningful addition to our family.

That evening I felt an overwhelming presence of peace fill my heart. Although I was still broken, I actually felt like I could move forward knowing that my baby was in a much sweeter place, and we would always have our angel watching over us. From that day forward I knew I would never look at a monarch butterfly the same.

The following week was hard. I was trying to sort out all of my emotions while trying to go back to my day-to-day responsibilities. I would cry to songs on the radio or when I saw a baby or a pregnant mother. Sometimes I would just cry. My husband would often ask what was wrong, and all I could ever tell him was "nothing but the obvious." It seemed to me that he was already over it. I often got upset with how he was dealing with our loss. I felt like it was no big deal to him once we had the service. It was not until I got a package from a friend back in Pennsylvania that included many poems and songs that helped her through a loss the year before that I really stepped back and looked at how this had affected my husband. One poem in particular that stuck out to me was one entitled "A Father's Grief." I cried for a long time after reading the words in the poem. It explained how hard it is for a father to lose his child because people expected him to be strong and take care of the mother and often no one ever stopped to ask how he was doing. I ran to my husband with tears streaming down my face and apologized for being so insensitive to his feelings. I realized then that he too had lost his child, and although he was not grieving the same way that I was, he was hurting just the same.

I realized in the days following our loss how insensitive some people could be. People just didn't know what to say, and I would have preferred at times that they just not say anything. I was furious when people would tell me that it had happened for a reason or that I wouldn't have wanted a "messed up" baby anyway or that I was young and had plenty of time to have babies. There were people who were totally shocked to hear that we had had a memorial service for our baby. One person even said "Oh, do people do that?" To be honest, I don't know if people do that, but we did it, and we are glad we did.

People would tell me their stories of miscarriage and would tell me that they knew exactly how I felt. I know they were trying to relate, but for some reason that statement would make me mad every time I heard it. They may have suffered from a miscarriage, but they had no idea how "I" felt. I got a phone call from my grandmother in that first week, and she couldn't have said it better when she said, "Sarah, I can't say I know how you feel because we all deal with this sort of thing differently, but I can say that I know what it is like to lose a child both during pregnancy and after they are born, and I can relate to those feelings, and for that, I am sorry."

A whole week went by, and I was able to slowly get my life back in order. It was on Monday, July 19 that I was driving home from work and my cell phone rang showing an unknown number calling. Usually I do not answer these calls, but for some reason that day I did. I was unaware of the news I was about to be told. It was my obstetrician on the other line. She said she had some pretty bad and unexpected news to tell me. During our conversation I remember her telling me about the pathology results from my delivery. She said something about it showing that the pregnancy was actually a partial mole. I had no idea what she was talking about. In that split second I tried to think back to nursing school, and although I remembered hearing the term before, I for sure didn't remember what it meant. She went on to tell me I was going to need a lot of close monitoring for the next six months to a year, but I tuned her out after she used the words *cancer* and *chemotherapy*. My heart stopped for a moment as tears filled my eyes. "I am going to die," was all I could think. I dialed my mom's number after hanging up with the doctor while trying to maneuver to the side of the road. I was able to tell my mom through my hysterical cries what I had heard the doctor tell me. I know that what I said to my mom was not the most accurate information, but once I had heard the doctor use the "C" word I had lost sight of the rest of the conversation.

I continued my fifteen-minute drive home, although it felt like I was on the road forever. I could not wait to get inside the house and start Googling what it meant to have a "partial molar pregnancy." I wanted to make sure I knew as much information about it as possible before my husband and in-laws got home. I got all of the facts together so I could accurately tell them what I had been diagnosed with. What I found out scared me. Although the literature said that this type of "cancer" was very curable, I was upset with how rare it really was. I was afraid that my doctor was not going to know how to treat it, and I knew I needed to sit down and have a face-to-face conversation with her.

> **Thoughts From Grammy:** Life went on, and we were all working through the pain. Then my daughter-in-law got the call from the doctor that her pregnancy had been a partial mole. We had no idea what this was. When our Sarah educated us, we became consumed with not only the grief of the recent loss but also great concern for her health. The news of the possibility of the big "C" and concern about if she would be able to have a child in the future was overwhelming. Education and prayer are powerful. Support is essential.

The next day I had an appointment to get my labs done. I cried the entire time the phlebotomist was drawing my blood. I asked the obstetric nurse if I could possibly sit down and talk to the doctor. She let me know that the doctor was not in that day but told me to come in on Wednesday. When I finally got to sit down with my doctor, I could barely ask the questions that were running through my head. I wanted to know if there was something wrong with my husband or me that may have caused us to have this rare complication. She answered that it was just a fluke thing that happened during fertilization and that there was nothing anyone could have done to stop it from happening. She explained everything to me in detail. She told me I would have to have my blood drawn every week until my hCG levels were below 2. I would have to stay below 2 for three weeks in a row, and then we could move on to monthly blood draws for six months. She also told me that if my levels stopped dropping or started to go back up, that chemo was sometimes needed to help get the hCG back to normal. A sense of relief flooded my body when she told me that chemo was not commonly needed with a partial mole and was confident in saying that chemo was most likely not in my future. She then made it very clear that I was not to get pregnant until my hCG levels stayed below 2 for six consecutive months, because it would make it too hard to tell if the molar cells were growing back or if it was a viable pregnancy. She said I had to start birth control right away.

After hearing that comment, I was devastated. Although we were not planning on starting a family before we learned I was pregnant, the baby we lost had been very much wanted. After going through sixteen weeks of anticipation and having my hopes and dreams for our child torn away, my desire to be a mother was that much stronger. At that moment six months to a year sounded like an eternity. I also became scared that this mole was going to affect the possibility of having a "normal pregnancy." The doctor assured me that once we got through the next six months to a year that the molar would be behind me and I wouldn't have to worry about it in future pregnancies. While I was there, she asked me how the bleeding after the D&C had been. I told her that had I bled for only four days and had no bleeding at all for three days but that it started back up pretty heavily. She said that because the bleeding stopped and started up again that she was concerned that maybe there was some retained tissue. She wanted me to have another ultrasound and be scheduled for a second D&C if there was anything questionable seen.

I returned to the hospital the next day. I had blood drawn and then followed an ultrasound tech back to a room. It was not long before she told me that there was a visible mass and that it looked like I would need surgery again. She told me she would let my doctor know, and I was sent home. I had not even gotten out of the building when my phone rang. There was a nurse on the line calling to tell me that I was scheduled for a D&C in the morning. I was instructed to be there by eight o'clock.

We went through the same routine as before, although this time my husband's cousin took me to the hospital and my husband would be joining us when he got off work. It was kind of nice to spend some time with her. She had had a miscarriage eight years before and could relate to how I was feeling. I was not quite as nervous this time. I had the same nurse that I had had with my first procedure, and luckily, she remembered me and didn't ask any insensitive questions. While we were waiting in the preoperative room our pastor came to pray with us before they took me back. My doctor came in and told me that my labs showed that my hCG levels were at 2,525, and because we had never drawn my levels before the first D&C it was hard to tell what progress had been made. She explained that this time, because they knew it was molar cells they were dealing with, she would do a more aggressive procedure. She told me they would also use an ultrasound in the operating room to make sure all residual tissue was removed. She used the analogy of house cleaning to describe the need for a second D&C. I was told to think of the first procedure as a good house cleaning and the second one as a deep clean, as if trying to get the security deposit back when moving out of a rental, paying special attention to all of the small details. That made sense to me. After the procedure I was discharged with instructions to have my blood drawn the following Wednesday.

My husband and I talked about getting tattoos in memory of our baby. I already had two tattoos and was excited about the thought of getting one with such meaning. After a lot of thought I decided to get the miscarriage awareness ribbon with angel wings and the title of a poem that brought me some peace since my diagnosis: "Angels Never Die." I went to the tattoo shop on July 25 to see if the artist could put my thoughts into a design. I did not have plans on getting my tattoo that day but just wanted to get something drawn up. To my surprise the artist had no other appointments while I was there, and I left the shop with the most beautiful tattoo on my right foot. I loved the idea that my baby would always be "walking" with me!

I dreaded going into the doctor's office to have my blood drawn on July 27. It was just one more reminder of this horrible diagnosis. The actual act of having it drawn didn't bother me, it was the reason I was there that brought me to tears as the phlebotomist stuck the needle into my arm. She stopped and looked at me with concerned eyes questioning if I was okay. I let her know that she had done nothing wrong and to continue with what she was doing. She seemed a little hesitant, so I explained everything I had been through leading up to this blood draw. I left the office with a knot in my stomach. Now, I just had to wait for the results.

Electronic medical records made my waiting periods pretty easy. All I had to do was log onto my chart the next day, and I would have a message from my doctor with my results. My doctor's note read "Yeah, your hCG level is down to 173. Continue to check this weekly." I was amazed with the huge decrease in hormones and at that moment I had a small glimmer of hope.

Day to day I would often question how it was possible to miss someone so much without ever having the opportunity to meet them. Everywhere I went in the following weeks I felt like I was being punished. It seemed as though no matter where I looked I saw pregnant women or newborn babies. I remember one day in particular when I was waiting in line at Target. There was a teenage girl standing in front of me with her mother, and in the cart there was a baby girl sitting in her car seat. She was screaming, and the teenage girl walked over to tend to her. Right there in the middle of Target, tears started to roll down my face. After the teenager made a comment confirming that she in fact was the mother of that precious baby, I got ANGRY.

"Why, God?!" I thought. "Why did you bless that high school student who doesn't even look to be fifteen with a baby? Why did you take mine away from me? Why am I being punished? I am in a loving marriage and we wanted our baby. It may not have been planned, but we were ready to love our child. We were anxiously ready to give our baby a good home with two loving parents, but you took that away from us. Why? I bet that girl didn't even want that baby!" My anger grew as my mind was racing with questions. I tried to wipe the emotions from my face as it was my turn to pay for my things.

I walked to the car in a daze, and then I got mad at myself. "Who are you to judge?" I thought as the tears once again rolled down my cheeks. At that moment, I remembered something my mother would always say to me: "Everybody has a story." I kept repeating that in my head, but I couldn't help but think that there was no way anyone, much less a teenage girl, could have a story worse than mine. I was sure that that young mother could not have possibly felt pain like I was feeling at that moment. Yet again, something came over me and I began to apologize for all the mean things I had thought about that young mother, because it was true: I didn't know her story. I was just hurting and couldn't help but let the negative thoughts cloud my mind.

I had trouble logging onto Facebook after my diagnosis. It was hard to see all of the posts of pregnancy announcements and baby pictures while the only thing I could post was "This week is brought to you by the number..." There were days I would not even sign on because I was just not in the mood to cry.

Every week I had mixed feelings about going in for my blood draws. At first it was as if I was picking the scab off of a large wound every week when I sat in that phlebotomy chair. As time went on, week by week it slowly got easier. On August 3, I opened up my medical chart e-mail and read the note from my doctor that said "looking good, went down to 37," I could breathe a little easier. Then on August 10 it read "levels continue to fall appropriately, you are down to 18." August 17's note said "Looking good, 11. Continue to check next week." At this point, although I was happy every time I opened my chart, I felt a bit discouraged. At first my levels had dropped so quickly, but after a few weeks it seemed as though it was taking forever and only dropping by a few points. I kept reminding myself that we were at least moving in the right direction.

On August 26 my doctor said, "Continue weekly checks, almost back to normal. Your levels are at 7." I took a deep sigh after reading those words and cried. It felt like it had been so long since my life had felt "normal." I knew I was getting close, but in a weird sense it felt so far out of my reach. August 31 I was told to continue with my weekly checks; my hCG level was 5. I got the same message on September 7, with levels at 4. Then on September 14, my heart sank as I opened my chart and saw that my levels were at 4 for the second week in a row, and my note read, "Continue with another lab next week." I remembered my doctor telling me that I had to get to 2 to be considered normal and that if my levels stayed the same for three weeks in a row without a drop before getting to 2, chemotherapy may be needed. Again, I felt so close, but I worried that I would need drastic treatment for just two lousy little hCG "points." I asked everyone I knew to pray for me. At this point that was the only thing in our power we could do.

I was so nervous to go in for my labs on September 20 and terrified to check my mail the next day. To my surprise, however, although my levels were still 4, my note read, "You have had three normal hCG levels. Now you can test monthly for the next 6 months. Do your next draw in one month." I was in shock, thinking, "I thought she told me it had to be below 2. It is only at 4." I called the doctor's office. I didn't know what to think, but apparently either I had heard her wrong or she had misspoken when we were first discussing my treatment. She informed me over the phone that anything below 5 was considered normal, not 2 as I thought I remembered her saying. At that moment, I felt as though a huge weight were lifted off my chest. I could physically breathe easier. The past twelve weeks had felt like an eternity. My moods had changed in split seconds, going from sad to angry, frustrated, scared, hopeful, desperate, relieved—you name it, I had felt it at some point since my diagnosis.

> **Thoughts From Grammy:** Each week as the hCG number continued to reduce, we would give thanks and then pray that the next week they would continue to decline. These weeks and months were difficult for us; we knew it was brutal for them.

Over the next few months, the days got easier. I was having more good days than bad, and I smiled more than I cried. It was hard at times, but I was trying to acknowledge the thought that there was a reason why I had been diagnosed with a molar pregnancy, even if I did not quite understand. I became quite fond of butterflies, especially monarchs. I decorated my office at work with butterflies, and I smiled every time I would see one of the beautiful creatures flutter by me. Some days I would pray that on my way home from work I would see a butterfly. Even when it started to get cold in October and November I would long to see a monarch float by. Many days, I got exactly what I would ask for; to me, that was a sign that everything was going to be okay!

October is Pregnancy and Infant Loss Awareness Month, which many people do not know unless they have suffered the tragic loss of a child. I made a t-shirt to wear every Friday through October. It showed a pink and blue miscarriage ribbon that spelled "Hope," and on the back it said. "The angel in the book of life wrote down our baby's birth, she whispered as she closed the book, 'too beautiful for Earth.'" I was not going to suffer in silence like so many other people who had endured miscarriages. The pain of losing a baby is oh so real, regardless if we got to meet our babies or not. October 14 I had my first monthly blood draw, and I wasn't all that nervous. I had been sharing my story with so many people that I felt a bit at peace with everything that was going on. If people asked if I had any children I would just smile and say, "I have one in Heaven." Most of the time you could tell people were uneasy with that answer and did not know what to say. On October 16 we lit a candle at 7:00 p.m. along with many other families around the world who had suffered from the loss of a child.

November 14 was my second monthly blood draw. My hCG remained at 1. On November 25 I got my first period since being pregnant; I was probably more excited than I should have been. I know many women dread the week they are visited by "Aunt Flow," but I was relieved. This was my body's first step to getting back to normal and being able to house a future pregnancy.

As we approached December, all of my feelings of loss hit me. My due date was slowly approaching, and I was not sure how I was going to make it through Christmas. December 12 I had my third monthly draw, and still my hCG level was less than 1. By December 22 I didn't want to go to sleep because I was afraid of the mood I would be in when I awoke on my baby's due date. When I did wake on December 23, I had the worst uterine cramps I had ever experienced. I thought that life was playing a very cruel prank on me; on the day I should have been experiencing labor pains, I was enduring my second post-D&C period! I cried all morning and called my mom in disgust. As always, she said the most encouraging words and told me not to be upset but to be glad that my body was doing what it was supposed to do to prepare for a future pregnancy. She had me smiling at the thought of only two more monthly blood draws before we could try for the baby we longed for. I made it the rest of the day without crying. I was able to look at all of the butterflies in my office and smile at the hope they offered for my future. They were the symbol for our child, the symbol of transformation, the symbol of change.

For Christmas, instead of an angel or star at the top of the tree we placed a butterfly. We even included a butterfly in our family Christmas photo. From July 2011 on, a butterfly would always be a part of our family!

Thoughts From Grammy: There were ups and downs, but by the time the numbers were in the "safe" range, we were thankful for our daughter-in-law's health and were filled with the HOPE that we could someday answer the question "How many grandchildren do you have?" with, "One in heaven and one on Earth." That Christmas, the words HOPE were on our Christmas tree, and the butterfly was at the top. It always will be there as a reminder that we have a member of our family who has taught us so much about love.

I had my next set of labs drawn on January 13. Once again, my results were less than 1. I had just one more monthly blood draw before we would decide if we were going to actively try to get pregnant again. To my surprise, I didn't get my period on January 21 as I had expected. On January 23 I took a pregnancy test that came back negative. On January 26 my period still had not shown up, so I took another test. To my surprise, this time it came up positive. I got super excited at first, but then my excitement turned to terror as I wondered what my doctor would say. She had been so adamant that I not get pregnant until my hCG levels were negative for six months. I was afraid of what she would tell me to do. I got ready for work and never woke my husband to tell him my news. I was nervous. I confided in a friend at work because I was so torn. I questioned if I should keep it a secret, act surprised when my sixth and final blood draw came up positive, and tell my husband then? Or should I tell my husband now and call the doctor to let her know what had happened? I was so scared and had no idea what to do. We agreed that it was probably best to tell my husband and have him help make the decision about what to do from there.

When I got home from work I stuck a book called *My Boys Can Swim!* on my husband's pillow. We had discussed before that he would know I was pregnant if he found a book on his pillow. He knew exactly what my message was when he saw something on his pillow before he even read the title. Andrew was terrified. He was scared for my health. He insisted that I not wait and tell the doctor right away, so the next morning I called to make an appointment.

I talked to my doctor over the phone on January 27 and she told me I had to go in for an hCG check and schedule an ultrasound. On January 30 my hCG was 2,523. The doctor wanted me to go in every forty-eight hours for the next two weeks to look at the hCG trend. She said she was looking for the numbers to double every time to ensure a viable pregnancy. My early ultrasound showed the gestation sac and yolk with no questionable findings, so I was instructed to go back for a second ultrasound in two weeks. At that point they were estimating my due date to be September 28 based on my last period, which ironically had been December 23. I remember thinking to myself that everything happens for a reason. "How weird is it," I thought, "that this baby growing inside me has a due date based on my previous baby's due date? Although I did not have a baby in my arms, the baby in utero was going to be the same age as the baby I should be holding. To look back, I was so angry to be getting my period that day, and now look!" That thought alone brought me a little bit of comfort.

My numbers on February 1 were 4,983 going up on my third draw to 9,743. A note from my doctor read, "hCG numbers appear to be trending appropriately, and it appears to be a normal pregnancy. We will find out soon with the ultrasound!" My heart skipped a beat after reading her statement. I was extremely excited but scared all at the same time.

On February 25 I was eight weeks, five days pregnant, and I went in for my second ultrasound with my postmolar baby. The feeling I had when I saw that little heart flickering on the screen was indescribable. I had a lot of negative thoughts about all of the things that could still go wrong, but then I enjoyed the thought that I'd been given a "second chance" at motherhood. I had to consciously tell myself that I was allowed to embrace this new life, but I was so afraid of the "what ifs?" My doctor's note read, "Normal growth, everything looks good!"

At my next obstetric appointment I confided in my doctor about all of my worries and concerns about this pregnancy. She assured me that I could come into the office anytime I wanted to listen to the baby's heartbeat. She said she would let me have an ultrasound every two weeks until I was twenty weeks along to bring me a little "peace of mind." She told me that she did not expect that anything would go wrong and that my odds of having another mole were so low that she would not even consider me "high risk." I left her office with a glimmer of hope.

Our plans were to not tell anyone our news until I was at least sixteen weeks along and had made it further into this pregnancy than the last, but my body had other plans. I began to show pretty early on in my second pregnancy and had to share my news with the people I saw daily around twelve weeks because I had an obvious baby bump. I still had not told my family in Pennsylvania.

I went to the hospital for a routine ultrasound at fifteen weeks. I sat in the waiting room for what seemed like a lifetime and began to cry. My husband looked at me and asked what was wrong. I couldn't help but think that it had been at this ultrasound during the last pregnancy that we had gotten the horrific news that there was no longer a heartbeat. I was terrified that I would get the same news. The ultrasound technician was very sympathetic to my feelings when she took us back and made sure to point out the heartbeat as soon as she put the probe on my belly. What a relief.

Just a week later I injured my foot and had to wear a walking cast for six weeks. Only two days after wearing the cast I tripped on the deck while taking my dog out and fell face down while my dog dragged me down the stairs and across the yard. I stood up and didn't know what to think. I was covered in mud literally from head to toe. I walked into the house, and my mother-in-law looked at me and asked if I was okay. At that moment I started to cry. "I am okay," I told her, "but how do you ask the baby if it is okay?!" When I went in to change my clothes I noticed a red mark on my stomach, which indicated I had made some impact there when I fell. I planned to go to the doctor's office the next morning just to hear the baby's heartbeat, like the doctor had told me I could do at anytime. I figured that would give me peace of mind that everything was okay.

When I went to the office the nurse told me that she wanted me to see the doctor and explain my fall to her. My original obstetrician was not in that day, so I had to see someone new. I was nervous because this doctor did not know me, although she had my records in front of her. She did an exam and told me that I should have gone to the emergency department right after my fall. She explained that even if I felt fine, something could have happened to the baby. My heart sank. I was so worried that I was going to lose this baby too. I was devastated, although the doctor assured me that it was a good sign that I was not having any bleeding or cramps. They drew blood and said they would call me if I had to go in for a RhoGAM shot. I got a call a few hours later. They had found some of the baby's blood mixed with mine, which indicated that the baby had been injured in my fall. I needed to go back to the office right away. I returned crying, worried that I was going to get even more bad news. They gave me a shot and sent me to the hospital for further testing. I had a special ultrasound to look at the baby and to check to see how much blood actually had been lost. The doctor at the specialty clinic in the hospital told us that the blood loss was very minimal and appeared to have stopped, but he wanted to do another test in 2 days. He also informed us that at that time the baby was not anemic and everything still looked good.

I did a lot of praying at that moment. I just knew I would not be able to endure another loss. Two days passed, and we headed back to the hospital to recheck the baby for anemia and to have a level-two ultrasound done to check its growth. While we were there, we had the opportunity to get a really close look at our baby. It amazed me to see a little person moving around on that screen. It had ten little fingers and toes, the most precious little face, and a really strong heart. In the middle of our ultrasound we were asked if we wanted to know if we were having a boy or girl! I was super excited to be able to find out so soon. I was only sixteen weeks along, and my husband and I agreed that we would like her to put the results in an envelope for us. The doctor came in after the ultrasound and told us that our baby had not lost any more blood and was growing appropriately. He wanted us to return in two weeks just to be sure.

We were ecstatic to see our baby thriving! We agreed that we wanted to have a gender reveal party with our close family and friends and have them all find out if we were having a boy or girl with us. We planned the party for the next day and dropped the envelope off at the bakery. Our request was to have a white cake iced with pink and blue polka dots, with the center icing being pink or blue based on what was in the envelope. The baker was thrilled to be a part of our surprise. The next day we had friends and family meet at a local coffee shop for the reveal. We had my family in Pennsylvania on Skype as we cut into the cake to find…BLUE icing! We were having a boy!

Our next specialty appointment confirmed that our baby was still growing appropriately and that there did not appear to be any residual effects from my fall. The doctor told us that based on the tests and ultrasound, our baby was going to be healthy, with no Down syndrome or any heart defects. He said our baby boy was measuring on track to be just less than seven pounds. I could breathe again. Within the next few weeks I was able to feel my little guy moving around more and more! It was such an amazing feeling. I was able to enjoy my pregnancy with the constant reminders from my little boy's kicks that he was still alive and well. I no longer questioned every symptom. I came to love being pregnant. I looked forward to every single one of my appointments and loved to hear my doctor tell us of our progress. It became real! I was actually going to have a baby.

My husband and I traveled home to Pennsylvania to see my family in July. My mother planned a baby shower for me while I was home. I woke up on the day of my baby shower and was getting ready when it dawned on me. It was exactly 1 year ago that day that I had gone to the hospital to have my first D&C. I cried as I was washing my hair. I thought of how happy I should be to be celebrating the life of the baby I was carrying, but yet I mourned for the baby I had lost the year before. During all of the planning of the baby shower, I never even realized that it was planned on the one-year anniversary of my molar pregnancy journey. Once again, I was reminded that everything happens for a reason. It was nice to be surrounded by all of my friends and family celebrating the new life I would be delivering in just a few months. It forced me not to sit around and mope over the traumatic loss I had endured. Still, after everyone left, I lit a candle and cried. I talked to my belly and told my son the significance of the date. I remembered my angel baby and gave my belly a light squeeze!

My son's due date came and went, and I had to be induced eight days late. Although I was feeling wonderful and never really minded being pregnant, I was ready to meet my rainbow baby. While I was in labor the nurses monitored me closely and at one time had trouble finding my son's heartbeat. I broke down and cried. At that moment I feared the worst. I looked at the nurse as tears streamed down my face and pleaded with her. "Please, I cannot lose him now." Her response was, "Don't worry sweetheart, we won't let that happen."

Seventeen hours after being induced, I got to meet my sweet baby boy. Bradyn Liam joined our family on October 7, 2012, weighing in at 6.15 pounds and measuring 21 inches long. As soon as I saw him, I was filled with an overwhelming amount of love that I had never thought possible. I thought I had already felt so much for this little miracle, but I was shocked to find that my love was so much more than I had anticipated. I don't even know how to describe it! While looking at that precious little boy in my arms I whispered, "You were definitely worth the wait!"

Thoughts From Grammy: The day came when we found out there was another pregnancy. Again, the pure JOY of a grandchild, but then the horrible worry over our daughter-in-law's health and the health of the baby. After nine months of her and our son's journey, I was there to welcome into the world our beautiful Bradyn Liam. One day, I will tell him about his sister in heaven looking down on him and praying for him and his family, the sister we will all get to meet some day when our time here on Earth is through.

During this whole journey I became stronger than I had ever thought possible. I could not even mention the incident without tears when I was first diagnosed, but the more people asked me about it and the more I talked about it, the easier it got. Slowly I was able to tell my story without tears. I would even smile at times with a sense of empowerment. By the time I graduated from weekly to monthly blood draws, I was eager to tell people what I was going through with the hope of educating them about the tragic misfortune of molar pregnancies. At some point along the way, and I am not quite sure when, I was given peace about our loss. I am not saying that the peace replaced all bad days, because it did not. What it did was allow me to have more good days than bad, and I know that even if the reason was not completely clear to me, there *was* a reason I had to go through all of the suffering that came along with my molar pregnancy. I have had a few people thank me for being so open about the loss of our child and acknowledging its existence, because it gave them reassurance that it was okay to grieve the loss of their own miscarriages. That alone may be why I had to endure the hardest thing any parent would have to do—to let go and say goodbye.

My son has not taken the place of my first baby. I still think of my molar baby as my first child. I think of that baby often and still cry when I imagine what could have been. I know I would not have Bradyn if I had not lost the first baby, but I can't help but wonder how my life would have been different. I feel guilty at times when I cry over the baby I lost while holding the most perfect little guy in my arms. My angel baby will always be a part of my life, and one day when Bradyn is old enough to understand, we will tell him about his sibling who we never got to meet. For now, I cherish every moment I have with my rainbow, and I smile as I watch the butterflies in the wild!

*For the beauty of a rainbow does not negate
the ravages of the storm. When a rainbow appears, it doesn't mean the storm never happened
or that the family is not still dealing with its aftermath. What it means is that something beautiful and full of light has appeared in the midst
of the darkness and clouds. Storm clouds may
still hover but the rainbow provides a counter-
balance of color, energy and hope.*

— Author unknown, answering the
question, "What is a rainbow baby?"

Simone

My husband and I went on holiday to New Zealand with friends. I was about eight weeks pregnant, and the holiday and my pregnancy started out happily. We visited the tourist attractions, and one of the tours was on a boat. At one point the boat went over a wave and gained a little air. I landed heavily on my seat and felt a gush of liquid come out. I shrugged off the feeling and told myself that I must have imagined it. When we got back to our apartment, I checked my underwear and found I had started lightly bleeding. The blood was brown and only a small amount. I told myself not to panic and remembered what my doctor had told me earlier in the year when I had miscarried. Brown is good, because it is old blood. I breathed a sigh of relief and informed my husband. We tried not to get too concerned and enjoy our holiday. The following few days I did bleed red blood, but it was only small amounts. Again I remembered my doctor saying if I don't soak through a pad, I will be fine. The bleeding stopped a few days later. I pushed the thought from my mind because I *felt* pregnant. Every morning I woke feeling queasy, and I had a constant hunger and tiredness.

A few weeks later I had my first antenatal appointment at approximately ten weeks. The visit was routine, and I received two ultrasound referrals, one for the genetic testing and one for the dating scan. That afternoon I booked the dating scan and had my blood tests. The following day I phoned to confirm the hCG levels and that I was pregnant. My levels had come back at 380,000. I became excited. My levels during my previous pregnancy had been below 1,500 at eight weeks, and that pregnancy had ended in miscarriage. I thought 380,000 must be better. My inquisitive side got the best of me, and I turned to my good friend Google and researched normal hCG levels in pregnancy. My levels were much higher than normal. I continued to read down the page, and it listed possible reasons. My dates could be wrong—not likely, this was our first month not using protection. Multiple babies—scary thought, but also exciting.

The last possibility was molar pregnancy. What was a molar pregnancy? Over the following two days I researched and read for hours, day and night, educating myself about possible reasons to explain what could be happening. I did not fit into the category for a molar pregnancy because I was younger than forty, had not had multiple miscarriages, and did not have a vitamin A deficiency. Two symptoms stood out: brown spotting and extreme pregnancy systems. At that moment I thought that I might not be pregnant after all.

A few days later my husband and I attended our ultrasound. I lay quietly on the table as the ultrasound technician applied warm gel to my stomach. I stared at her as I waited, looking for a glimmer of hope. Her forehead was creased and her lips pressed together. Minutes went by. She started to shake her head and said, "This does not look good." I instantly burst into tears and knew it was all over. The technician turned the screen, which showed the large mass of shapes. She began explaining what I was seeing, but she did not have to say a word. I already knew as much as she did. She excused herself and informed my doctor. We left the room and waited to see him.

I tried to pull myself together and looked around to see if I knew anyone in the waiting room. I quickly realized it was the free immunization clinic, and I was surrounded by what felt like all of the newborn babies who lived in my town. I looked back down at my hands. I could not tell you how long I sat there. Seconds felt like minutes, and minutes like hours. I could not breathe. I got up, walked around the corner, and started crying. My name was called, and I entered the doctor's office, where he told me the molar tissue was large and I could not have the operation performed in my local hospital because I needed two bags of blood on hand just in case. He arranged an appointment with the specialist who would perform the operation and told me that I was not allowed to fall pregnant for one year.

The following day I saw the specialist. He was warm and made me feel comfortable. He scheduled my surgery for his next available date, two days later. He explained the possible complications, including scarring, puncturing, hemorrhaging, and worst of all, hysterectomy. He also said that if my hCG levels decreased without needing further treatment, I would only have to wait six months before I could try again. I felt that my body had failed me and I would never have a baby. My pregnancy had ended the moment the ultrasound technician had started shaking her head. I wanted the operation over and my body back without missing organs. The following day I had a chest X-ray just to make sure the molar tissue had not spread; fortunately it was clear.

We drove to the hospital early Friday morning. On the way there I wished the car ride would not end, that we would escape reality and drive away from our current situation. Reality sank in when my husband parked our car and we made our way into the hospital. I changed into my hospital gown and disposable underwear. I inserted two tablets high into my vagina to start dilation and sat down next to my husband in the waiting room as the cramping started. I felt a sigh of relief that it was going to be over soon. My name was called, and I hugged and kissed my husband but did not want to leave him. I wished he could have been by my side through the operation, because when he is with me I feel safe. I lay down in the hospital bed and the nurse covered me with warm blankets. Then I was wheeled off into operating theater. My last thoughts were, "Please let me wake up, please let me keep my uterus and have a baby one day."

What felt like moments later I woke up. I felt my stomach and it seemed normal, but the disposable underwear had been removed. In its place was a large absorbent sheet. I breathed a sigh of relief. The theater nurse met with me shortly after in recovery. The operation had gone well, and no blood was required. I got dressed and was picked up by my eagerly waiting husband. We left the hospital and drove home to start the recovery process.

Recovering from a molar pregnancy is physically hard, but emotionally it is much worse. I cried many times a day for weeks. I felt as though I had failed to become a mother and had let down my husband, friends, and family. I did not want to go out in public, because I had failed at the most basic process of life. I thought I would be judged because I could not become a mother. As my hCG levels dropped I started to feel better. I would not cry as much, and eventually if I did not cry for one day I classed that as a positive day.

I had my weekly blood test on Friday mornings because I believed that I could not worry over the weekend, and this routine helped me relax. Every Monday morning I phoned the medical center for my results.

It was Monday morning, and I was relaxing in bed reading the news. My phone started to ring, and it was the medical center. My stomach dropped, and I watched it ring for a few more seconds. When I answered, it was my doctor. He quickly got to the point: my hCG level from the previous Friday had increased by ten points to 660. I could not respond. He said I had to get an ultrasound, and he wanted me to wait and see if the rise in hCG was due to a laboratory error or something else. The phone call ended, and I lay down on my bed and imagined the molar cells traveling through my blood to my organs.

Thirty minutes later the phone rang again. This time it was my specialist who performed the surgery. He had spoken to the oncologist and my doctor, and they also had agreed to wait and see what my next blood test results showed.

Wednesday afternoon I felt cramping in my lower abdomen and had the urge to use the bathroom. I wiped myself and looked at the toilet paper. On the paper sat a piece of light pink tissue the size of a large grape. In the toilet bowel were two more identical pieces. The cramps went away, and I felt better. The following day I had the ultrasound and weekly blood test. The next day was Saturday, and my phone started ringing. I took a deep breath and answered. It was my doctor. I could tell by the excitement in his doctor's voice that it was good news. My blood level had fallen from 660 last week to 130. I was grinning from ear to ear as though I had just won the lottery. This was the best news I had received in a long time. The ultrasound had shown a small amount of tissue in my uterus, but my doctor believed that because of the dramatic drop in my hCG levels, the small amount of tissue was not a issue. A few days later my period started, and although it was the worst period I have ever experienced, I was excited to finally have it again. It was heavy, with lots of cramps, but I felt that my body was getting back to normal. My blood test results dropped from 130 to 63, then 63 to 10, and 10 to 0.

After two more test results at 0, I started on monthly blood tests. My poor arms were thankful for the break. I had blood tests every month for six months, and during that time I focused on my health and becoming as fit and healthy as I could be. I started to run and eat a balanced diet. I took vitamins, fish oil, and coenzyme q10 so I could prepare my body to the best of my ability to one day have a baby. I attended the last blood test filled with a mix of emotions. I was happy that this chapter of my life was coming to a conclusion, but I was also scared of the unknown and the fear of another molar pregnancy. That day I completed my Pandora charm bracelet by purchasing a die to remember that day. The die represents life and reminds me that sometimes life is a gamble. My husband and I celebrated the end of the blood test and my molar pregnancy that night by going to dinner. We drank wine and spoke about the future together and what it may hold.

My due date for my molar pregnancy was quickly approaching, and I was unsure if I should acknowledge the date or pretend as though it had never existed. I made the decision to not acknowledge my due date and successfully managed to wipe the exact date from my memory. We also were told that my husband's brother and his wife were expecting their first child. I was very excited for them but broke down in tears. I was not jealous, but I felt that it was never going to be my turn and that I would never have a baby. Shortly afterward I knew that I wanted to try for another baby. Little did I know that I would conceive in the following few days!

Two weeks later my period was late, but I shrugged it off because my cycle was never perfect. Three days passed and my period was still a no show. My nipples were hard, which attracted the attention of my husband; he gave them a playful tweak and they started to leak. We looked at each other and said nothing, but I knew I was pregnant. Two days later I took a pregnancy test and held my breath and shut my eyes. Minutes later I opened them, and two lines were clearly visible. I walked outside and showed my husband. "Don't get your hopes up," he said. I booked myself in for an early doctor's appointment and ultrasound.

On the day of the ultrasound I was overwhelmed with fear. I was on the verge of being sick and crying. I lay down on and table and the ultrasound technician applied the warm gel. I lay still and stared at the ceiling until I heard the technician say, "We only have one baby." I instantly had tears streaming down my face and said, "We have a baby." I felt like a kid at Christmas time, and I looked over to my husband. He was grinning from ear to ear and had tears in his eyes. We were pregnant with a baby that was 12 mm long and had a healthy heartbeat. The ultrasound technician played the heartbeat over the speakers, and I stared at the screen in amazement. I had a tiny life growing inside of me. I would like to say that the fear of something going wrong disappeared that day, but it didn't. Throughout my pregnancy I believed the doctor was going to tell me bad news. Every blood test or ultrasound, I prepared myself for the worst. Shortly after the ultrasound I purchased a Doppler so I could listen to my baby's heartbeat at home, and I listened at least once a day until I felt constant movement. Whenever I listened to the baby's heartbeat I felt calm and re-assured that I was still pregnant.

The fear finally disappeared on the January 22, 2013 at 10:17 p.m., when I held my beautiful baby girl for the first time. I now know that life is truly amazing. If I had to have a miscarriage and molar pregnancy as part of the process to give birth to my daughter, I would. When I was pregnant in 2011 for the first time I wanted a boy. With the second pregnancy, the molar pregnancy, I did not care if I had a boy or a girl. When I fell pregnant again at last in 2012, all I wanted was a healthy baby. What sex I preferred was not a consideration. Now that I am finally a mother, I don't take the role for granted. I believe if I had not had the pregnancy losses I would not appreciate the role of a mother as much. I have had to work hard physically and mentally to get where I am today, and I will never think that pregnancy and parenting is just a way of life but rather, a true blessing. I would not have gotten through this process without the love and support from my family, friends, and doctor. This experience has strengthened the relationship I have with my husband; he held me while I cried in pain, sorrow, and joy and kept me focused on reality and what matters in life.

"I believe everything happens for a reason.
Things go wrong so that you can appreciate
them when they go right and sometimes good
things fall apart so better things can fall
together."

— Marilyn Monroe

hCG Levels

- Pre-D&C: 380,000
- 1 week after D&C: 4,600
- 2 weeks after D&C: 795
- 3 weeks after D&C: 650
- 4 weeks after D&C: 660
- 5 weeks after D&C: 130
- 6 weeks after D&C: 63
- 7 weeks after D&C: 10
- 8 weeks after D&C: 0

Stacey

Back in June of 2011, my husband and I made the decision to see a fertility and reproductive endocrinology specialist to help us get pregnant again after I was diagnosed with polycystic ovarian syndrome (PCOS). My irregular cycles had been making it difficult, and we thought by seeking help, we would soon become pregnant. Meanwhile, my OB/GYN had given me Clomid to take to see if it would work. To our surprise, when I underwent the ultrasound, we saw that I was about to ovulate and that there was, in fact, an egg "ready to go." The doctor instructed us to "get busy," and wished us luck.

We had just moved into our new home, and many friends and family had sent us blessings, including a lot of "new house, new baby" comments. We wanted more than anything for that to be true. Our son Jack, who was three years old at the time, was asking for a sibling often, and we were ready to get pregnant. A week after our fourth wedding anniversary in July, I found out I was pregnant. After months of frustrations, we did it (figuratively and literally)! As soon as I could, I called my OB/GYN's office and was schedule for an eighth-week appointment in early August. In the meantime, I began to have that "Oh my God, I'm pregnant!" excitement. I began dreaming about life with a new baby and entering a new chapter in our lives.

My appointment could not come soon enough; we were so anxious. We knew my dates were right, because I had been on Clomid and had charted everything since my last period, but the ultrasound only showed a sac, nothing else. The heartbreaking reality of a miscarriage began to overcome me. I was told to wait it out a week or so, and if I did not miscarry on my own, I would have to have a D&C. I went home and cried and cried. Instead of wanting the baby so badly, I wanted to miscarry and get it over with. It was a surreal feeling. I knew what was inside me was empty and that the sooner it was gone, the sooner I could move on. Days went by. I agonized at night and suffered from mid-night sleeplessness. After a week, we made our appointment to have the D&C.

The only time I had ever been to the hospital before was to have a baby, and now I was there to lose what was supposed to be one, or wasn't one to begin with. I was told that while I was under, they were going to do a pathology test to make sure the cells were removed. When I woke up, I was informed that all had gone well, but that the cells were abnormal. They were XYY and considered a chromosomal abnormality typically associated with a molar pregnancy. I remember saying, "What does that mean? Why? What is that?" over and over again. I thought I'd feel relief, but instead I felt fear.

I soon learned what a molar pregnancy was. I remember, as they were explaining it, wondering if it was gone and what if it comes back?, but I was made to feel that the D&C had been thorough and I was in the clear. They were to monitor me with weekly blood draws to make sure my hCG beta levels continued to go down. Apprehensive still, I felt that if my doctors were confident, I should be too. So I salvaged what little time I had left of the summer before work and school started and tried to be happy and think about moving on.

You know you have a problem when you go to the local laboratory facility so much that they now "know you." This is exactly how I was beginning to feel. I had been going for so much lab work that I was officially a "regular." My levels were monitored and continued to drop, but not as quickly as I thought they would. No one at my OB/GYN's office had told me my results were abnormal, so I didn't worry, but on Columbus Day, in the middle of a workshop I was attending with fellow educators, I got the call that changed my life.

It was the tone of the nurse's voice that immediately struck me. It just sounded like she was about to give me bad news. She had called to inform me that my levels had gone up, not down, and that this was highly concerning. There were only two possibilities: one, I was pregnant (but clearly couldn't be) or two, the mole had come back or never fully had gone away. I was asked to come to the office to sit down and discuss options. With a lump in my throat, I called my husband and then immediately went to the office.

I have always trusted my OB/GYN and thought that his care was exceptional. Now I felt leery. Was this his fault? Was it mine? Everything went through my mind in the car on the way there. The look on my face must've said it all; the first words out of his mouth were, "Calm down, everything is going to be fine." In my mind, though, it wasn't fine. WHEN, WHEN would it be fine? I felt like I had suffered so much already, and I just did not think I could emotionally or physically handle any more. I was informed that the recommended course of treatment would be injections of a drug called methotrexate. Okay, that didn't sound so bad. "When can I start taking it?" I asked. As it turned out, methotrexate is a chemotherapy drug, and I would have to see a gynecologic oncologist first. In my head I was now screaming, "WHAT?! ONCOLOGIST?!" When you hear the news that you have to see an oncologist, the first thing you think is cancer, right? I was now more freaked out. On top of it all, I wondered how this would affect my future ability to conceive again. Would I ever be able to have a baby after all this?

There were so many other things happening my life, like making sure my son was taken care of or would be when I wasn't feeling well and that things at work would be okay without me. I hated knowing I was going to have to use a lot of sick days so early in the year, but I convinced myself that I HAD to make myself a priority. It felt as though the weight of the world were on my shoulders, and I was overwhelmed.

I remember sitting in the waiting room of the oncologist's office looking around at the other patients and thinking about what they must be going through. I thought I should stop feeling so bad for myself; they probably had it so much worse than me. But I couldn't stop. I was scared and anxious and frustrated. Why me? My husband and I met with the doctor and were told that there were two types of molar pregnancies, partial and complete. As I had had no fetus, they were leaning more toward my issue being a complete mole. Regardless, the treatment was the same. Before I could undergo the injection of the methotrexate I would need another trip to the laboratory and a CT scan of my lungs and ultrasound of abdomen to ensure that none of the diseased cells had spread. Hello, more anxiety! "What happens if the cells do spread?" I asked, and I was sorry I had. I was told that treatment would be more severe and result in a stronger form of chemotherapy that would likely lead to hair loss and other symptoms. Before we left with our pile of scripts in hand, I wanted to know what this meant for our future fertility. I was thankful to learn that despite the immediate chaos, I would be able to get pregnant in six to twelve months after completion of treatment. At least I had that.

I immediately set up my exams and appointments and then went home, where I had nightmares about the "What ifs." Time seemed to move too slow for me while I awaited results and clearance on how to proceed. Fortunately everything came back "normal," and I was set up to undergo the first round of methotrexate.

When you go to the hospital and have to check-in in their "cancer center," you have an out-of-body experience. Why am I here? How did this happen to me? Why me? Not knowing what I was going to have to endure, I had my awesomely supportive husband come with me. He had been my rock through this all, traveling to and from work long distances to meet up and accompanying me through appointments and testing, and today, I really needed him to hold my hand. As we entered the infusion center I saw people in beds and in chairs with IVs in their arms. They looked miserable and sick, and I felt this awful feeling in the pit of my stomach. Yet I wanted to be here, I wanted to get this "thing" out of me and move on.

As it turned out, my injection would not be intravenous, but given intramuscularly through my lower back (yeah, in my butt) in two shots. This way it is a slow release and more effective. So after yet another blood draw and a dosage of Zofran (to help with side effects of nausea and dizziness), I literally dropped my drawers and held my breath.

In the days after, I felt sick on and off. It was as though I had a perpetual cold that didn't want to go away. The worst part was that I could not have any alcohol—so I couldn't have that glass of wine I so badly wanted to help me relax! It killed me. Follow-up was blood work, again, and anxiously awaiting results to see if it worked. I remember checking my phone in my pocket every five minutes. Did I have it vibrating? Is the ringer loud enough? I just wanted to hear some good news for once! When they did finally call, they said that it was working, but not well enough. I would have to go again. I felt crushed, sick, and panicked. Again? Could I handle doing this AGAIN? When I came home, my adorable little boy looked at me and asked, "Mommy what's wrong? You need to feel better." I knew I had to do it again. I had to get past this. I had to get well again, even if it meant feeling worse first.

So yet another round of lab work and another round of methotrexate. I did not know what to expect this time; would the side effects be worse? Will this be it? I was an emotional basket case! This time the side effects hit me harder. I had to miss yet another day of work just to stay home and recuperate. I couldn't get out of bed and just prayed this was it. The day I went in for my follow-up blood work I purposely went early in the morning and then went to work to help distract myself.

Finally, at the end of the day, I got the call. This time, for the first time in months, the voice at the other end of the phone sounded perky and happy. I took a deep breath. "So tell me, what are my numbers like?" I couldn't contain my excitement and joy when the nurse said that my numbers were great and that I would not need to go again. I let out tears and could not wipe the smile off my face. FINALLY, for the first time in months, some good news! My numbers were going down.

Of course, it wasn't totally over. The levels got "stuck" at 30 for a couple of weeks, and I had to undergo the worst of it all: daily small-dose injections for 1 week. It didn't bother me at first, but the aftermath was horrible: nausea, mouth sores, overall feeling awful. I even ended up having to take a trip to the local emergency department to get some intravenous fluids into me. However, my numbers were now so low they were barely undetectable.

Once my levels were officially "normal," I had to undergo one more dosage. This time I was prepared mentally and physically for the side effects and aftermath but was at peace knowing that this was IT! After the long and draining road, I was looking forward to getting rid of the mouth sores, destroyed tummy (which required weeks of medicine to heal), lethargy, and constant tearing eyes. There would still be weekly blood draws for a few weeks and future testing to ensure that my numbers continued to stay normal, but I looked forward to happy times and feeling well and knew that in the future our family would grow—just not right now. I was okay with that.

One of the biggest things I realized through all of this was what fabulous team of doctors I truly had and how fortunate I was.

I became pregnant as soon as I was cleared to try again in July 2012. As I write this I am at twenty-six weeks. We are due with our second boy, our postmolar baby, in March 2013. The pregnancy road after a molar is not easy, and it was hard to enjoy the many joys the way I did the first time around. I was filled with anxiety and nerves constantly and even still today. Yet despite all the anxiety, I'm excited and overjoyed that our family will be growing soon and that my body was able to give me another baby after all the drama was said and done.

Appendix: Web Sites and Support Groups

Web Sites

MyMolarPregnancy.com
http://www.mymolarpregnancy.com

This is my Web site, founded in 2001. The site includes information and links related to molar pregnancy, a support group, and additional personal stories.

About.com Pregnancy/Birth: Molar Pregnancy
http://pregnancy.about.com/od/cancerinpregnanc/a/
 Molar-Pregnancy.htm

American Cancer Society:
Gestational Trophoblastic Disease
http://www.cancer.org/cancer/
 gestationaltrophoblasticdisease/index

American Pregnancy Association: Molar Pregnancy
http://www.americanpregnancy.org/
 pregnancycomplications/molarpregnancy.html

BabyCenter: Molar Pregnancy
http://www.babycenter.com/0_molar-pregnancy_1363614.bc

BabyZone: Understanding Molar Pregnancy
http://www.babyzone.com/pregnancy/
 pregnancy-complications/molar-pregnancy_78812

Band Back Together: Molar Pregnancy Resources
http://bandbacktogether.com/Molar-Pregnancy-Resources

Charing Cross Hospital Trophoblastic Disease Service
http://www.hmole-chorio.org.uk

Cleveland Clinic Health: Gestational Trophoblastic Tumor
http://my.clevelandclinic.org/health/diseases_conditions/
    hic_Gestational_Trophoblastic_Tumor

Dana Farber Cancer Institute:
Gestational Trophoblastic Tumor
http://www.dana-farber.org/Adult-Care/Treatment-and-Sup-
    port/Gestational-Trophoblastic-Tumor.aspx

Eyes On the Prize: GTD Stories
http://www.eyesontheprize.org/stories/dx.html#gtd

Feedback: A Pro-Life Doctor's View on
Molar Pregnancies (Answers in Genesis)
http://www.answersingenesis.org/articles/2012/05/18/
    feedback-pro-life-doctor-molar-pregnancies

Foundation for Women's Cancer
http://www.foundationforwomenscancer.org

Grief Loss & Recovery
http://www.grieflossrecovery.com

Gyncancer.com: Gestational Trophoblastic Disease
http://www.gyncancer.com/gest.html

HAND: Helping After Neonatal Death
http://www.handonline.org

Hannah's Prayer: Christian Support for Fertility Challenges
http://www.hannah.org

HopeXchange
http://www.hopexchange.com

Hygeia Foundation
http://hygeiafoundation.org

Intelihealth (Harvard): Molar Pregnancy
http://www.intelihealth.com/article/molar-pregnancy

International Society for the Study of Trophoblastic Diseases
http://www.isstd.org/index.html

Lab Tests Online: hCG Tests
http://www.labtestsonline.org/understanding/
    analytes/hCG/glance.html

March of Dimes: Ectopic and Molar Pregnancy
http://www.marchofdimes.org/loss/molar-pregnancy.aspx

Mary Stolfa Cancer Foundation: Gestational Trophoblastic Tumor
http://marystolfacancerfoundation.org/
    GestationalTrophoblasticTumors.html

Mayo Clinic Online: Molar Pregnancy
http://www.mayoclinic.org/diseases-conditions/
    molar-pregnancy/basics/definition/con-20034413

Medline Plus: Hydatidiform Mole
http://www.nlm.nih.gov/medlineplus/ency/article/
    000909.htm

Memorial Sloan-Kettering Cancer Center:
Gestational Trophoblastic Disease
http://www.mskcc.org/mskcc/html/1909.cfm

Miscarriage Support Auckland
http://www.miscarriagesupport.org.nz/molar.html

MolarPregnancy.co.uk: Comprehensive U.K. site
offering information, guidance, and support forum
http://molarpregnancy.co.uk/index.html

National Cancer Institute:
Gestational Trophoblastic Tumors
http://www.cancer.gov/cancertopics/pdq/treatment/
    gestationaltrophoblastic/Patient

Oncolink: University of Pennsylvania Cancer Center
http://www.oncolink.org/experts/
    article.cfm?id=1647&aid=2647

"Presentation and Management of Molar Pregnancy"
(Book Chapter)
http://www.isstd.org/isstd/chapter09_files/GTD3RDCH09.pdf

Silent Grief
http://www.silentgrief.com/

Unspoken Grief: Signs and Symptoms
of Ectopic and Molar Pregnancy
http://unspokengrief.com/signs-and-symptoms-of-ectopic-
    and-molar-pregnancy/

What to Expect: Molar Pregnancy
http://www.whattoexpect.com/pregnancy/
    pregnancy-health/complications/molar-pregnancy.aspx

Wikipedia: Molar Pregnancy
http://en.wikipedia.org/wiki/Molar_pregnancy

YouTube: Molar Pregnancy
http://youtu.be/LcZbuc8raOQ

YouTube: What Is a Molar Pregnancy?
http://youtu.be/bprrUG6i3pM

Support Groups

MyMolarPregnancy Support Group
https://www.facebook.com/groups/mymolarpregnancy/
*Private Facebook-based support group for women recently diagnosed
or currently going through treatment for molar pregnancy or
choriocarcinoma.*

After My Molar Pregnancy Support Group
https://www.facebook.com/groups/aftermymolarpregnancy
*Private Facebook-based support group for women cleared to conceive
after a molar pregnancy or choriocarcinoma (or at least ready to
talk about trying again; this group can be difficult for those still
dealing with the initial grief of the molar miscarriage, as it does
involve discussion of conception, pregnancy, and birth after molar
pregnancy, so please be aware before requesting membership).*

Glossary

beta qual: Blood test that detects pregnancy based on the quality of the hCG in a blood sample. This is the blood test normally done when a pregnancy is suspected. It indicates the presence of elevated hCG but does not give a specific amount of hCG.

beta quant: Blood test used to detect the exact amount of hCG in women with gestational trophoblastic neoplasia. This test is used for nonroutine detection of hCG. "Normal" levels of hCG are generally considered to be levels less than 5, although this varies among physicians and facilities.

chemotherapy: The use of chemical agents to kill cancer cells or stop them from growing. These agents can be given intravenously, intramuscularly, or orally, depending on the drug being used.

choriocarcinoma: Cancerous form of gestational trophoblastic neoplasia that develops in placental tissue in the uterus and may metastasize to other parts of the body. It can occur after a normal pregnancy, miscarriage, ectopic pregnancy, or genital tumor but most often occurs with a complete molar pregnancy. Usually curable if caught early enough and treated aggressively with chemotherapy; however, it can recur within a few months to as long as 3 years after treatment. Choriocarcinoma is much more difficult to cure if it has spread or other factors are present; consult your physician for more information.

dilation and curettage, D&C: A minor procedure in which the cervix is expanded enough to permit the cervical canal and the lining of the uterus to be scraped with an instrument known as a curette. This procedure is sometimes done after a miscarriage or during an abortion.

dilation and evacuation, D&E: Although essentially the same procedure as a D&C, a D&E is most often done for second-trimester miscarriages or abortions and uses more vacuum evacuation and requires more cervical dilation because of the larger quantity of tissue removed.

ectopic pregnancy: Pregnancy in which the fertilized egg implants not in the uterus but in the fallopian tube, ovary, or abdominal cavity. This is a serious condition and must be treated quickly.

gestational trophoblastic disease (GTD; also known as gestational trophoblastic neoplasia, GTN): An "umbrella" term for any condition due to abnormal tissue growth composed of trophoblastic cells. Normally, this tissue is supposed to connect the zygote (fertilized egg) to the uterine wall and to help form the placenta. The two main types of GTD are hydatidiform mole (molar pregnancy) and choriocarcinoma.

human chorionic gonadotropin, hCG: Hormone produced by the placenta that is detected by blood and urine pregnancy tests to indicate a pregnancy. hCG levels are affected by molar tissue; thus this hormone is used as an indicator for possible regrowth after a molar pregnancy.

hydatidiform mole: An abnormal growth of the membrane that encloses the embryo and gives rise to the placenta. If a mole develops, the embryo is usually either absent or dead. The mole itself is a collection of cysts that contain a jellylike substance and resemble a cluster of grapes. These cysts can grow very large if not removed, but most are removed by D&C. In a few cases, the mole can spread into the uterine muscle and cause bleeding. In very rare cases these moles can develop into choriocarcinoma.

intramuscular, IM: Used to describe an injection in the muscle, such as the shoulder, hip, or buttock.

intravenous, IV: This term literally means "in the vein." The abbreviation is also used as a noun to refer to an intravenous line used to administer fluids.

invasive mole: Molar tissue that grows and spreads into and beyond the uterus, possibly metastasizing to other areas of the body.

molar pregnancy: An abnormality of the placenta caused by a problem when the egg and sperm join together at fertilization. A *complete molar pregnancy* occurs when sperm fertilizes an empty egg. No baby is formed, but placental tissue develops. The placenta grows rapidly and produces elevated hCG levels. A *partial molar pregnancy* occurs when two sperm fertilize the same egg. The fetus, which has too many chromosomes, usually dies in the uterus. Again, unusually high hCG levels are usually an indication.

peripherally inserted central catheter (PICC): A thin tube used to give medicine such as chemotherapy over a period of time; the tub is inserted in the arm or chest into a vein.

persistent mole: Molar tissue that regrows or continues to grow after the D&C. A second D&C may be performed before, or in addition to, treatment with chemotherapy.

ultrasound, abdominal: A painless, noninvasive procedure in which sound waves are used to produce images of the inside of the body. Reflected sound waves are received by instruments called transducers, which are small, handheld devices that are moved back and forth across a patient's abdomen to form an image. A lubricating gel placed on the abdomen helps facilitate movement of the transducer.

ultrasound, vaginal: A form of ultrasound in which special probes are inserted into the vagina to obtain better images of a fetus or other uterine condition.

Made in United States
Orlando, FL
19 May 2022

18005807R00138